W9-CFF-922

Instructor's Manual with Test Bank to Accompany

Critical Care Nursing: A Holistic Approach

Sixth Edition

Carolyn M. Hudak, PhD, RN

Nurse Practitioner
Denver, Colorado

Barbara M. Gallo, RN, MS, CNAA

Assistant Professor
University of Hartford
School of Education, Nursing, and Health Professions
Division of Nursing
Hartford, Connecticut

Test Questions Written By:

Anda Craven, RN, MS, CCRN

Assistant Professor of Nursing
Oregon Institute of Technology
Klamath Falls, Oregon

Barbara Krumbach, RN, MS, CCRN

Clinical Educator, Surgical ICU and Burn Unit
University Hospital
University of Colorado Health Sciences Center
Denver, Colorado

Kathleen S. Oman, RN, MS

Clinical Nurse Specialist
Surgery/Trauma Service
Denver General Hospital
Denver, Colorado

J. B. Lippincott Company

Philadelphia   Hagerstown

Sponsoring Editor: Diane Schweisguth

Editorial Assistant: Sarah L. Andrus

Compositor: Richard Hartley

Ancillary Coordinator: Doris Wray

Printer/Binder: Capitol City Press

0-397-55118-5

7 6 5 4 3 2 1

Any procedure or practice described in this book should be applied by the health-care practitioner
under appropriate supervision in accordance with professional standards of care used with regard to
the unique circumstances that apply in each practice situation. Care has been taken to confirm the
accuracy of information presented and to describe generally accepted practices. However, the
authors, editors and publisher cannot accept any responsibility for errors or omissions or for
consequences from application of the information in this book and make no warranty, express or
implied, with respect to the contents of the book.

Every effort has been made to ensure drug selections and dosages are in accordance with current
recommendations and practice. Because of ongoing research, changes in government regulations and
the constant flow of information on drug therapy, reactions and interactions, the reader is cautioned
to check the package insert for each drug for indications, dosages, warnings and precautions,
particularly if the drug is new or infrequently used.

Table of Contents

CHAPTER 1

> # *Integrating Nursing Process and Nursing Diagnoses Within a Holistic Framework*

CHAPTER OUTLINE

Behavioral Objectives

Description

Integrating Nursing Process and Nursing Diagnoses in Critical Care

Nursing Diagnoses

Steps in the Nursing Process

Holistic Framework

Hierarchy of Human Needs

Promoting Adaptation

The Critical Care Nurse as Advocate

Study Questions

BEHAVIORAL OBJECTIVES

Based on the content in this chapter, the reader should be able to:

1. List four issues influencing current critical care nursing practice.

2. Define nursing diagnoses.

3. Outline the steps of the nursing process in critical care nursing practice.

4. Briefly describe how the principles inherent in Maslow's hierarchy of human needs can serve as a holistic framework for critical care nursing.

5. Describe the concept of adaptation.

6. Describe three specific nursing actions that foster adaptive functioning in the critically ill patient.

OVERVIEW

Chapter one presents a framework for providing nursing care in the critical care unit. The steps of the nursing process and formulating nursing diagnoses are described. Concepts which are discussed include Maslow's hierarchy of human needs, promoting adaptation, fostering security, and serving as a patient advocate.

KEY TERMS

nursing process	hierarchy of human needs
nursing diagnosis	
adaptation	nurse as patient advocate

TEACHING/CLINICAL STRATEGIES

1. As part of clinical experience have student formulate nursing diagnoses and develop nursing care plans.

2. Have students discuss the care planning (nursing) process for their patients

throughout their clinical experiences.

3. In clinical conference ask students to identify their nursing interventions to increase their patients' sense of security (trust).

TEST QUESTIONS

1. One of the major issues facing the critical care nurse today is:
   A. simpler technology
   B. increasing younger population
   • C. ethical dilemmas
   D. decrease in health care costs

2. Nursing diagnoses are identified by using the:
   • A. nursing process
   B. patient bill of rights
   C. a code of ethics
   D. nightingale pledge

3. Mrs. H. complains of pain in her left lower back. The first step in the nursing process for the nurse would be to:
   A. decide that the pain is coming from a muscular area
   B. administer morphine
   C. ignore the complaint as Mrs. H. is always complaining
   • D. perform a pain assessment

4. Which of the following statements is true about critical care nursing?
   A. the essence of critical care nursing lies only in special environments
   • B. the essence of critical care nursing is based in a decision making process that lies in a sound understanding of physiological and psychological entities
   C. the essence of critical care nursing deals only with all the special equipment they must deal with
   D. critical care nurses deal critically with only one body symptom at a time

5. Alteration in cardiac output related to an acute myocardial infarction is considered:
   A. a plan of care
   B. an intervention
   • C. a nursing diagnosis
   D. a psychological assessment

6. Which of the following statements is true regarding nursing diagnosis?
   A. they address only physiological and psychological problems in health
   • B. based on a nursing diagnosis, the nurse can independently initiate interventions to solve the problem
   C. they reflect medical responses to potential health care problems
   D. reflect only actual problems

7. The first step of the nursing process includes:
   A. planning an intervention
   B. stating an expected outcome
   C. re-evaluating the plan
   • D. collection of subjective and objective data

8. Providing adequate fluids is a:
   A. nursing diagnosis
   • B. nursing intervention
   C. part of an initial assessment
   D. medical diagnosis

9. Mr. T. is complaining of shortness of breath. An outcome criteria based on the plan of care can be stated as:
   A. oxygen administered
   B. instruct the patient to take deep breaths
   • C. the patient will be able to breathe comfortably while lying flat
   D. raise the head of the bed

10. Steps in the nursing process are:
    • A. assessment planning, implementation, and evaluation
    B. planning and evaluation
    C. assessment, planning, writing a nursing diagnosis
    D. assessment and evaluation

11. The most basic needs in Maslow's Hierarchy are aimed at:
- A. self preservation
  B. security
  C. self-worth
  D. belonging

12. Physiological amputation refers to:
  A. removal of a limb
  B. a decompensated state
- C. directing energy away from less critical functions in order to help an organism through a physiological crisis
  D. maintaining upper level needs such as self-esteem

13. Adaptation is defined as:
  A. fleeing from a situation
  B. the body's defenses destroying the stressor
- C. retaining a steady state while seeking to establish a compatible response to stress
  D. assessing and intervening in a stressful situation

14. Mr. B. has been admitted with complaints of chest pain. He does not want to report episodes to the nurse because he wants to go to his son's graduation. She talks to him about the need for reporting the pain and helps him discover ways to interact with his son for graduation. The nurse's response is an example of:
- A. adaptive nursing intervention
  B. avoidance
  C. counteraction
  D. maladaptive nursing intervention

15. Which of the following actions describes a nurse's effort in the role of a patient advocate when a look of fear occurs on the face of a patient who is intubated?
- A. speaking directly to the patient while explaining nursing care
  B. keep his hands always restrained so he won't pull out his ET tube
  C. talk to MD about patient's care while ignoring his expression
  D. discuss upcoming staff meeting with peer while caring for the patient

CHAPTER **2**

Psychosocial Concepts and the Patient's Experience with Critical Illness

BEHAVIORAL OBJECTIVES

Based on the content in this chapter, the reader should be able to:

1. Describe the relationship between stress and anxiety.

2. List the behavioral and physiological symptoms of anxiety.

3. Identify and describe methods to increase a patient's sense of control and reduce a sense of helplessness.

4. Describe three methods of assisting patients in coping with anxiety.

5. Identify and describe the stages of grieving and describe nursing interventions for each stage.

6. Discuss a nursing intervention that fosters the ability of patients to draw strength from their personal spirituality.

7. Describe the phenomena of transference and countertransference as they occur in

critical care nursing.

8. Describe appropriate interventions for transference and countertransference.

9. Discuss the emotional implications of transferring a patient from the critical unit and describe interventions that will assist the patient in coping with changes.

OVERVIEW

Chapter 2 presents concepts aimed at supporting patients and families through the stress of crisis and adaptation related to illness or death. Anxiety, dependency, and response to loss are described along with nursing measures that support patients through these stressors. Some of the measures described are internal dialogue, guided imagery, and relaxation. Nursing actions which increase the patient's sense of control and foster constructive responses are also described.

The four stages of response to loss are explored along with nursing actions which foster adaptation. Spirituality and its healing influence are explained along with the need for nurses to acknowledge an individual's beliefs and values. Content on adaptation to illness discusses the nurse's responsibility for evaluating the patient's response to illness in order to support effective behaviors and redirect ineffective behaviors.

Transference and countertransference are also explained along with suggestions for coping. The last issue examined is preparing the patient and family for transfer from the CCU. Factors to consider include the timing in relation to the patient's physical and emotional response to the critical illness.

KEY TERMS

coping	internal dialogue
disequilibrium	external dialogue
denial	mental imagery
anxiety	transference
dependence	countertransference
cognitive techniques	

TEACHING/CLINICAL STRATEGIES

1. Have students practice internal dialogue (self-talk) and relaxation techniques in order to gain experience and confidence before helping a patient or family member use them. (See Exercises that follow.)

2. Have students identify two behaviors that they find hard to deal with, how they feel, and the way in which they usually respond.

3. In conference have students discuss their patients' physical and psychosocial responses to illness as reflected in patient behaviors.

EXERCISES FOR QUESTION 1

Each of us experiences anxiety in our lives. The following techniques are designed to lessen anxiety. Try them out on yourself in order to gain experience and confidence before helping a patient or family member use them.

a. Focus on your "self-talk" or internal dialogue. Does it concern a problem that troubles you? Does this dialogue increase your anxiety? Does it contain thoughts that are negative about yourself? If so, say these thoughts out loud to yourself. Think about what you have said and concentrate on changing parts of this self-conversation so that it is more positive and realistic. If, for example you are worried about an upcoming event, pare the event into bite-sized pieces. then focus on achieving each one, step by step. Changing what you say to yourself can control anxiety.

b. Try out the following relaxation exercise.
   - Pick a quiet place where you can lie down.
   - Take several deep breaths and let them out slowly.
   - Let your body sink into the couch or mattress so that all body parts are supported.
   - Start the muscle tensing and relaxing with your toes and work up toward your head.
   - Start by curling your toes as tightly as possible.
   - Hold that position for a few seconds and then let go.
   - Feel the sensation as your toes unclench.
   - Then, point your toes up toward your head as far as possible. You will feel your calf muscles tighten.
   - Then relax your feet and savor the sensation.
   - Next, tighten your thigh muscles by pressing the back of your knees into the couch.
   - Hold the position for a few seconds and then relax your knees.
   - Continue this process of tensing and relaxing your muscles with your buttocks, abdomen, fingers, upper arms, and shoulders.

- Take a few deep breaths and let them out slowly as you go along.

- Imagine the tension draining out of your body as you relax.

As you concentrate on the muscle relaxation, your mind will clear of thoughts.

Before sitting up, enjoy your relaxed feeling for a few moments.

TEST QUESTIONS

1. Admission of a patient to a critical care unit:
   A. allows a patient to feel safe and secure
   - B. may cause a patient to perceive his admission as a sign of impending death
   C. may cause a patient to realize he has to take control of his life
   D. allows the patient to openly communicate with the nurses his feelings

2. A state of disequilibrium or tension that prompts attempts at coping is considered to be a state of:
   A. anger
   B. denial
   - C. anxiety
   D. stress

3. A physiological response to stress could be:
   A. dry skin
   B. constricted pupils
   C. slightly decreased blood pressure
   - D. rapid pulse rate

4. A person who is concerned about getting better asks "Am I going to die?" The nurse replies "You'll be alright." He may feel a sense of:
   A. regression
   - B. isolation
   C. comfort
   D. anger

5. Mr. O. is confined to bed and experiencing a sense of loss of control. The nurse might:
- A. include him in small decisions
  B. reduce the number of visitors
  C. tell him that he will be okay
  D. decide for him the best place to put personal items

6. A patient admitted to a ICU may be heard to say "I can't stand it in here." This is an example of:
- A. internal dialogue
  B. external dialogue
  C. feeling a sense of isolation
  D. feeling a sense of loss of control

7. A patient states to the nurse "I can't do anything for myself." This is an example of:
- A. external dialogue
  B. internal dialogue
  C. fear of dying
  D. a sense of isolation

8. During progressive relaxation a patient:
- A. relaxes one group of muscles at time
  B. talks feelings out loud
  C. imagines being in a strange place
  D. makes his own choice

9. The best way for the nurse to cope with an overly dependent patient would be to:
  A. say "I've got other patients to take care of."
- B. tell the patient when she will return
  C. avoid the patient because he is too demanding
  D. tell the patient that he will be okay without her being in the room

10. Mr. Z. has been told that he has suffered an acute myocardial infarction. He says to the nurse "I just had indigestion." This is an example of:
  A. awareness
  B. restitution
  C. resolution

- D. denial

11. The best way to help a patient in the anger/awareness stage is to:
  A. say that you feel sorry for him
  B. say that he should not feel that way
  C. state "getting mad at me won't help."
- D. provide the need for privacy and ventilation of feelings

12. During the phase of restitution, the patient may:
- A. reminisce about the loss
  B. try to go home
  C. blame the nurses for everything that has happened
  D. feel guilty about what has happened

13. While assisting a family during the stage of restitution, the nurse may:
  A. tell the family that they will just have to accept what has happened
  B. encourage them not to discuss their feelings with the patient
  C. tell them they should not be feeling the way they are
- D. allow the family to ventilate their feelings

14. Transference occurs when:
  A. the nurse becomes angry with the patient because he will not do as told
- B. the patient says to the nurse "you just don't care".
  C. the patient states "I just want to die".
  D. the patient states "I can handle this pain if I do it one step at a time".

15. When a patient is transferred from the critical care unit, the nurse should:
  A. ignore the termination process because of the quick need to move
  B. tell the patient that he is moving immediately before he does
- C. explain the transfer process in advance
  D. expect the patient to handle the process okay because he is getting better

CHAPTER 3

Caring for the Patient's Family

Behavioral Objectives

Based on the content in this chapter, the reader should be able to:

1. Identify and describe the characteristics of a crisis event.

2. Identify variables that determine the meaning of crisis events for patients and family members.

3. Identify goals that assist families in coping with crises.

4. Describe the nurse's role in a helping relationship during times of crisis.

5. Identify and describe nursing behaviors in assisting families coping with crises.

6. Identify and describe nursing goals and behaviors associated with caring for dying patients and their families.

OVERVIEW

Chapter 3 explores the ways in which families try to maintain equilibrium even in the face of crisis. Four generalizations are presented which form a basis for the nursing care of families. Principles include establishing an emotionally meaningful relationship and helping the family define the crises and its meaning, see alternatives, and define steps they can take. The next section describes how nurses can care for families when the patient is dying. Listening, being consistent, and fostering equanimity are some aspects of care. Near death experiences are also described because of the increasing numbers of people who survive and remember them. Nurses can assist patients and family members by acknowledging the importance and meaning of the experience to them.

KEY TERMS

family	cognitive mastery
cognitive appraisal	family integration
biological crisis	out of body experience
emotional crisis	

TEACHING/CLINICAL STRATEGIES

1. In conference have students respond to the following situations by identifying the feelings the family members are experiencing.

   a. The parents of a terminally ill son repeatedly plead to the nurse, "We want the best, no matter what it costs." The nurse might say, "You feel ...

   b. A patient is being transferred to a medical unit and the family responds angrily by saying, "She's not ready to be moved. Can't you see that she still has IVs in her?" The nurse might say, "You feel ...

   c. Family members are asked to leave the bedside of a patient and the family responds by saying, "You allow the Smiths to stay constantly with their father." The nurse might say, "You feel ...

   d. The family members continuously advise the nurses regarding the small details of patient care.

   e. A patient has died after a short but acute illness. Family members become hysterical and accuse the nurses by saying, "Why didn't you take better care of him? Why wasn't someone with him?" The nurse might say, "You feel ...

2. Have students role play the following situations with each other, taking turns and switching roles. Have them give feedback to one another about the specific responses. A psychiatric-mental health nurse specialist may join the group for facilitation or consultation.

   a. RJ is a 30 year old patient with AIDS who has an advance directive for no CPR. Because RJ's condition has deteriorated and he is not expected to survive this episode of PCP, the physician has addressed withholding CPR with the family and SO, RJ's best friend. SO tearfully tells you that he cannot believe that this is really the end.

   b. There is little hope that a patient will survive. He must be transferred to a private room on a medical unit in order to make room for a new admission to the critical care unit. The family has been in the waiting room around the clock for three days. Although the physician has told them of the patient's prognosis, you must notify the family of the impending transfer.

   c. A nurse returns from her coffee break by way of the waiting room. She learns from family members of the patients that someone has had a cardiac arrest, and all family members were asked to leave. The families' anxiety appears to be contagious. Some people are pacing while others are talking loudly or crying. Each person seems to believe that it is his relative who is near death. Everyone begins to converge on the nurse asking "Who has had a cardiac arrest?"

TEST QUESTIONS

1. When a family member is admitted to a critical care unit, the family:
   - • A. may exhibit an emotional crisis
   - B. always group together and accept the situation
   - C. exhibit adaptive behavior
   - D. are always able to make clear decisions and mobilize resources on their own

2. When first meeting the patient's family, the nurse should:
   - A. state that everything will be okay
   - • B. explain equipment and what is going on
   - C. rush in and out because she has to see another patient
   - D. expect that if the family is coping now, they will surely cope later on as well

3. Patients that describe floating above their own bodies or seeing dead family members:
   - A. need to have their pain medication lightened
   - B. need a psychiatric consult
   - C. always die shortly thereafter
   - • D. may be experiencing a near death experience

4. When a patient enters the critical care unit, the nurse must realize that:
   - • A. the contributions of the hospitalized person may be lost to the family
   - B. the patient is the only concern and the needs of the family will have to be dealt with by someone else
   - C. the family gather together to fulfill the missing role
   - D. all families will react the same

5. A family crisis occurs when:
   - A. the present state of family equilibrium is maintained
   - B. the usual problem solving activities are adequate
   - C. the family is able to carry the social, but not the financial, role of the patient
   - • D. a stressful event occurs and threatens lasting changes for the family

6. The following is true of a crisis:
   - A. what is crisis for one family, is a crisis for another
   - • B. stressful situations that have occurred prior to the current even have an impact on the current situation
   - C. families assign the same catastrophic meaning to the same events
   - D. the quality of help during a crisis has no impact on whether family members emerge stronger

7. When a critical care nurse deals with a family crisis, she should first:
   - A. work with the patient and not think of the family
   - B. tell the family that the doctor will tell them everything
   - • C. assess the immediate events causing the disruption and help the family assign priorities
   - D. disregard their feelings because it is the patient who is most important

8. Defining the immediate problem in a crisis situation
   - A. is not helpful
   - B. increases anxiety in the family members
   - • C. helps family members assign priorities that need action
   - D. does not assist the family in understanding what is happening

9. The process of helping the family view a problem from a different perspective is called:

10

- A. reframing
  B. coping
  C. cognitive mastery
  D. assessment

10. When a family is faced with a crisis, the nurse can:
    A. help them to rely on themselves and not others
  - B. research how they handled stress before
    C. tell them that they must contain their own feelings
    D. make all their decisions for them

11. When a nurse assists a family to focus on expressing their reactions and starts a statement with "you feel", she is reflecting:
    A. a problem
  - B. a feeling
    C. a judgement
    D. a decision

12. During the process of problem solving, the nurse should:
    A. deal with the problem herself and not involve others
    B. give small meaningless advice to make the patient feel better
  - C. focus on the here and now and not on previous long term problems
    D. emphasize only the patient's concerns

13. When a patient dies, the nurse should:
    A. not show any concern
    B. keep her thoughts to herself
  - C. demonstrate comfortably concerned compassion
    D. feel she has failed in her duties

14. When keeping a patient who is near death comfortable, the nurse should:
  - A. consider pain relief as an important part of that comfort
    B. not over medicate for fear of addiction
    C. ignore the patient's desire to be alert even if somewhat uncomfortable
    D. express feelings that men should be able to handle pain better than women

15. During the time the patient is dying, the nurse should:
    A. always be sad and solemn
    B. avoid allowing children in for fear of upsetting them
  - C. expect complaints and criticism towards her
    D. keep strict visiting hours

CHAPTER **4**

Psychosocial Impact of the Critical Care Environment

BEHAVIORAL OBJECTIVES

Based on the content in this chapter, the reader should be able to:

1. List five factors which may adversely affect patients in the critical care unit.

2. Identify five nursing interventions which can minimize the effects of sensory deprivation and sensory overload.

3. Explain how periodicity affects the patient in the critical care environment.

4. Discuss potential problems caused by sleep deprivation.

5. List ten possible causes of acute confusion.

6. Identify five nursing interventions which encourage reality orientation.

7. Identify actions which acknowledge the patient's need for personal space and privacy.

OVERVIEW

This chapter covers a range of factors that can adversely effect patients in critical care units.

The first concept discussed is sensory input which includes sensory overload and sensory deprivation and their effects on critically ill patients. The assessment section describes evaluating the critical care environment and the patient's response to it, and tailoring nursing interventions based on the nursing history. The management section explores actions aimed at minimizing the quantity, while improving the quality, of sensory input. Ways to provide meaningful information to confused and unresponsive patients and suggestions for limiting noise are discussed.

Next, the stages of sleep and the consequences of sleep deprivation are presented. Nursing responsibilities for ensuring adequate periods of uninterrupted sleep are discussed. Last, acute confusion and its potential exacerbation in critical care units are presented. The precipitating factors, symptoms, assessment skills and management are described. Nursing actions that foster reality orientation and preserve personal boundaries are included.

KEY TERMS

sensory overload

sensory deprivation

informational
underload

perceptual
deprivation

sensory restriction

periodicity

Slow Wave sleep

Rapid Eye
Movement sleep

circadian rhythm

TEACHING/CLINICAL STRATEGIES

1. Have students evaluate the type and amount of sensory input in the critical care unit to which they are assigned. Discuss in conference.

2. Have students choose a patient they can

interview and gather information from the patient, chart, and staff about the amount and description of the patient's sleep for a 24-48 hour period. Discuss in class or conference.

3. Arrange a presentation with patient examples on acute confusion conducted by a geriatric nurse specialist.

4. Have student(s) evaluate the medication and other factors which may contribute to sensory overload and deprivation for an elderly patient in critical care. Discuss in conference.

5. Have student(s) observe an unresponsive patient for two hours and record the sensory input (sights, sounds, activities, verbal and nonverbal communication including touch). Discuss in conference.

TEST QUESTIONS

1. The critical care nurse should realize that:
   A. patients admitted to critical care units maintain normal coping defenses
   B. patients can handle sensory overload better than sensory deprivation
   • C. patients frequently fear the technology in the CCU
   D. technology is important and will not have an adverse affect on the patient

2. The following is true of sensory impact:
   A. too much of a stimulus is not the same as too little
   • B. individual perceptions of stimuli vary from person to person
   C. patients in critical care environments do have control over too much stimuli
   D. quality not quantity of stimuli is important to consider

3. Loss of sense of time, boredom, depression, psychosis, can be symptoms of:
   A. sensory overload

- B. sensory deprivation
  C. personal lack of space
  D. state of denial

4. Symptoms of decreased hearing, panic, confusion, and delusions can indicate:
   - A. sensory overload
   B. sensory deprivation
   C. fear of dying
   D. sensory restriction

5. The hospital phenomenon refers to:
   A. bland tasting food from dietary
   B. visits by a multitude of health care professionals
   C. lack of privacy and control over environment
   - D. a combination of sensory deprivation and sensory overload

6. Bright lights, monitor alarms, ventilator noises and loud voices can contribute to:
   - A. sensory overload
   B. sensory deprivation
   C. hospital phenomenon
   D. poor self-esteem

7. A continuous input of familiar meaningful information from the patient's outside world refers to:
   A. sleep deprivation
   B. sensory deprivation
   C. sensory overload
   - D. reality testing

8. Those most susceptible to sensory deprivation are:
   A. females
   B. males
   - C. those who are unconscious
   D. middle aged patients

9. The planning of care for an unresponsive patient might include:
   A. constantly changing nurses caring for the patient

- B. standing very quiet at the bedside
- C. playing the patients favorite music
  D. discouraging family members from touching the patient

10. Providing information about time, date, year and explanation of procedures to a patient with an altered state of consciousness can provide :
    - A. security information
    B. nothing
    C. an increase in sensory deprivation
    D. an increase in sensory overload

11. A decrease in noise level, decrease in light intensity, controlling environmental odors, and tactile communication can decrease:
    A. depression
    B. sensory deprivation
    C. sleep deprivation
    - D. sensory overload

12. Mental restoration occurs during which stage of the sleep cycle:
    - A. stage I - sleep latency
    B. stage II - delta sleep
    C. stage III - REM latency
    D. stage IV - REM sleep

13. Which of the following actions provide for adequate REM sleep?
    A. bathe patient between 2 a.m. and 5 a.m.
    - B. increase visiting hours during non-sleep periods
    C. routinely take vital signs every 1-2 hours
    D. continue all nursing care activities regardless of the time of day

14. Nursing interventions for a patient who is confused include:
    A. avoid touching the patient
    B. keep curtain open so patient can be seen at all times
    - C. provide meaningful sensory stimulation
    D. plan nursing care activities in the early morning hours

15. Entering a room before knocking or taking pictures of loved ones from the bedstand without permission, can have an effect on one's:

- A. need for personal space
  B. need for sensory stimulation
  C. need for reality testing
  D. need for decrease in sensory overload

CHAPTER 5

The Dynamics of Touch in Patient Care

CHAPTER OUTLINE

BEHAVIORAL OBJECTIVES

Based on the content in this chapter, the reader should be able to:

1. Discuss the concept of caring and how it is used through touch behaviors in nursing.

2. Identify messages sent and responses to touch as described in nursing literature.

3. Delineate situations/factors that put patients at high risk for touch deficit.

4. List nursing assessment guidelines for evaluating touch needs of patients and families.

5. Implement the nursing process, including nursing diagnosis to address touch needs of patients.

6. Formulate a nursing care plan for patients threatened by touch deficit.

OVERVIEW

This chapter explores communicating with patients through the use of touch. After a review of the literature on caring and touch, the characteristics of touch are described: duration, location, frequency, intensity, and sensation. A taxonomy explains the 5 levels of touch beginning with level 1, functional/professional. Patients and families at risk for touch deficiency are described and include those with sensory deprivation, body boundary threats, fear, anxiety, loss of control, separation and communication barriers. Assessment guidelines are included and nursing management is illustrated in a case study and nursing care plan.

KEY TERMS
taxonomy of touch   hypohugganemia

TEACHING/CLINICAL STRATEGIES

1. Have students write about the implications for touch by responding to the situations listed under Exercises for Question 1. Discuss in conference.

2. In conference have students discuss their individual style and reaction to level 1, function/professional touch.

3. In nursing lab have students role play the situations described under Exercises for Question 3 in which touch can be used supportively along with verbal communication.

EXERCISES FOR QUESTION 1

Now that you have an increased understanding of the qualitative symbols of touch behaviors, describe how your increased awareness of their effects can have implications on patient care. Identify possible implications for each of the following situations *in relation to specific qualities of touch identified*.

1. Mrs. G. is an 84-year-old widow who was admitted this morning at 10:00 a.m. via ambulance. She was found weak and confused lying on her living room floor. It is suspected that she suffered a stroke.

    a. What are the implications in regard to *intensity* of touch?
    b. What are the implications in regard to the *duration* of touch?

2. Don, an 18-year old high-school athlete, has been in the critical care unit for 6 days. Last week he was traumatically injured while working on a new summer job in a factory. His left leg, left foot, and right hand were caught in a large machine. He has had extensive reconstructive surgery and hopes to regain full use of his leg and foot and partial use of his hand.

    a. What are the implications in regard to the *location* of touch?
    b. What are the implications in regard to

frequency of touch?

3. Mr. A., a 35-year old businessman, has been admitted to the ICU following a boating accident in which he suffered multiple lacerations and contusions, a mild concussion, and severe fractures of both legs. He is in constant, severe pain and asks for analgesics frequently.

   a. What are the implications in regard to the *sensation* of touch?
   b. What are the implications in regard to the *action* of touch?

EXERCISES FOR QUESTION 3

With your classmates, use role playing to enact the following situations. Make an effort to use touch in a therapeutic and supportive manner in conjunction with effective verbal communication.

1. Mr. J. has been admitted to the ICU with acute pulmonary edema. He is restless, short of breath, and frightened. You are his nurse.

2. You are the charge nurse in the ICU and one of your patients, Mr. B., has just returned from open heart surgery. You are going to bring his wife in to see him for the first time since surgery. You approach her in the waiting room.

3. Mrs. L. has been recovering from a severe episode of gram negative shock. She calls you to her bedside and, weeping, asks, ''Am I going to die?'

4. Miss S. is a 90-year old woman who was transferred to the ICU after an emergency colectomy. She seems to be recovering well from her surgery but has become increasingly confused and disoriented during the evening. After careful evaluation, you suspect sensory deprivation.

TEST QUESTIONS

1. Listening, respect for dignity, and sharing are important aspects of:
   A. technical nursing skill of nurses
   B. disease-oriented care
   C. communication
   • D. caring

2. Person-oriented care focuses on:
   A. pathology
   • B. quality of life of the patient
   C. illness
   D. preventative medicine

3. The need for touch is thought to intensify during:
   A. sleep deprivation
   B. sensory overload
   • C. episodes of high stress
   D. hallucinations

4. Nursing authorities agree that:
   • A. affective touch along with treatment-related touch can improve nurse-patient communication
   B. touch has no effect on physiological parameters
   C. touch conveys invasion of privacy
   D. the need for touch is only present in the elderly

5. Because of the increased likelihood of loneliness, touch is especially important in:
   A. males
   B. females
   • C. the elderly
   D. the middle-aged

6. A message conveyed by touch includes:
   • A. security
   B. invasion of privacy
   C. pain
   D. aloofness

7. The pressure used on the body surface during touch refers to:
   A. sensation of touch

- B. intensity of touch
  C. frequency of touch
  D. location of touch

8. According to Heslin's work, the nurse-patient relationship fits between which two levels of touch?
   A. level I - functional/professional and level II - social/polite
   B. level II - social/polite and level III - friendship/warmth
   C. level I only - functional/professional
- D. level I - functional/professional and level III - friendship/warmth

9. Hypohuggenemia refers to:
   A. advanced need of an adult
- B. a state of touching deficiency in a patient
   C. sensory deprivation
   D. advanced need of a child

10. The following statement is true about well-planned touch:
    A. is beneficial only with non-verbal communication
- B. enhances communication
    C. is only helpful in times of crisis

D. can be a barrier to communication when the patient is surrounded by machinery and tubes

11. Mrs. M. was involved in a motor vehicle accident. She was surrounded by tubes, machinery, nurses and doctors. The family was fearful of touching her for fear of disturbing the equipment. The following intervention might be utilized:
    A. keep strict visiting hours
    B. indicate that only the nurses should touch the patient
- C. demonstrate how to touch the patient without disturbing the equipment
    D. have the family stand only at the foot of the bed

12. In assessing the patient and family need for touch, the nurse must remember that:
    A. everyone reacts the same way to touch
- B. older patients have an increased need for touch during a crisis
    C. cultural practices do not affect the need for the amount of touch
    D. everyone needs the same amount of touch

CHAPTER 6

Patient and Family Teaching

BEHAVIORAL OBJECTIVES

Based on the content in this chapter, the reader should be able to:

1. Assess, carry out, and evaluate a patient teaching program.

2. Identify and describe a seven-step process for planning and carrying out a patient teaching plan of care.

3. Identify specific cognitive and psychomotor knowledge deficits and related patient goals and outcome criteria.

OVERVIEW

Chapter 6 explores the concepts of teaching and learning and applies them to the critically ill patient and the family. A seven step process is described for assessing the learner and designing and implementing a teaching plan. Motivation, knowledge level, readiness, resources, mutual goal setting, behavior change, and evaluation are explained. Concepts from other chapters such as adaptation to illness are integrated. Content is also included on developing nursing diagnoses, determining outcomes, and planning intervention. A sample teaching plan is included.

KEY TERMS

motivation	psychomotor change
knowledge gap	feedback
mutual goal setting	

TEACHING/CLINICAL STRATEGIES

1. In conference or class have students state whether or not they think the patients described below are ready for an increased

amount of learning and briefly give their reason.

   a. A patient has just been weaned from a respirator and still feels dyspneic.

   b. A patient states that she is feeling good physically and mentally and is looking forward to being transferred out of the critical care unit.

   c. A patient recovering from an auto accident is upset upon receiving the news that he has pneumonia and will have to remain in the critical care unit longer.

   d. A patient is very reluctant to admit that he has been critically ill.

   e. A patient who has been free of chest pain for several days is now receiving medication to ease chest pain.

2. In conference have students discuss how they would ensure that a patient received accurate information about the discharge regime when the patient is somewhat overwhelmed and fatigued by his impending discharge.

TEST QUESTIONS

1. Learning is most likely to occur:
   A. on admission to the critical care unit
  • B. during quiet stages when the emotional outlook corresponds with the physical condition
   C. right before discharges
   D. during transfer out of the critical care unit

2. Extrinsic motivation for learning includes the:
  • A. physical environment
   B. learner's attitude
   C. learner's personality
   D. learners's lifestyle

3. The nurse has more control over:

  • A. extrinsic sources of motivation
   B. intrinsic sources of motivation
   C. altering the patient's values
   D. altering the patient's personality

4. While assessing the knowledge gap the nurse should:
   A. assess knowledge in terms of "what could be"
   B. set goals for the patient, even if unrealistic
  • C. recognize what needs to be taught and learned in order to affect change
   D. realize that she has full control over what the patient will learn

5. During the steps of learning readiness, the nurse must:
   A. teach whenever it is convenient for her schedule
  • B. realize that worry, pain, and medications may interfere with a patients readiness to learn
   C. teach adolescents the same as adults
   D. expect the patient to remember everything told to him

6. To help insure patient learning the nurse may:
  • A. include pamphlets and booklets along with verbal backing
   B. expect the patient to remember everything told to him
   C. finish all teaching while in the hospital
   D. do all individual - not group teaching

7. During the teaching session, the nurse should:
   A. teach the patient everything
   B. state "this has happened to you, so you will learn about it"
   C. make the family remember everything that is taught
  • D. ask herself "Is what the patient and family wants to remember and learn, what I want to teach?"

8. When teaching, the nurse must:
  • A. assess availability of resources

B. set goals based only on her assessment of what is to be learned
C. teach only the patient
D. feel okay just to show videos without the opportunity for questions

9. A patient is to go on a low cholesterol diet. An appropriate teaching goal would be:
   A. the patient will have an understanding of all foods low in cholesterol
   B. the patient will list 25 foods low in cholesterol
   C. the patient will list all foods to avoid
   - D. the patient will be able to list 12 foods low in cholesterol by the time of discharge

10. Which of the following teaching techniques would be most effective in getting a patient to stop smoking?
    A. telling him he must do it by himself
    B. telling him that his wife demand that he quits
    - C. developing a teaching plan that includes reinforcement and encouragement
    D. encouraging the patient to do it for his family

11. A patient must lose 50 pounds. He has lost 5 pounds. Appropriate feedback would be:
    - A. you lost 5 pounds; great
    B. you'll die if you don't lose the rest of your weight
    C. you'll hurt your family if you don't lose it
    D. you're doing good, but not good enough

12. The most appropriate way to assess if a patient has learned how to draw up insulin, would be to:
    - A. have him demonstrate drawing it up
    B. have him state how it is to be done
    C. give him a written test
    D. check in nurses notes to see if he was taught

13. Utilizing the affective domain one deals with:
    A. evaluating the learner's ability to perform a certain procedure
    - B. the clarification of the patient's values and beliefs
    C. referral process after discharge
    D. ability to communicate how to do the procedure

CHAPTER 7

The Critically Ill Elderly Patient

BEHAVIORAL OBJECTIVES

Based on the content in this chapter, the reader should be able to:

1. Identify ten physical changes occurring as a result of the normal aging process.

2. Identify the developmental tasks of the elderly.

3. Describe prevalent conditions which affect the major body systems of the elderly.

4. Discuss age-adjusted parameters for the elderly.

5. Describe why the principle *start low, go slow* is important for the elderly in regard to the absorption, distribution, metabolism, and excretion of medications.

6. Formulate a nursing care plan, using the nursing diagnosis format, for the gerontologic patient.

OVERVIEW

Chapter 7 presents the biological, developmental and psychosocial issues that accompany the later phases of aging. Physical, psychological and medication assessment are covered. Changes associated with aging are examined for each body system (including sensory and sleep). Three guiding considerations include: (1) a change in one organ or system does not predict changes in others; (2) changes cannot be chronically predicted because of wide variations; (3) changes due to disease must be distinguished from changes associated with aging. The psychological assessment discusses cognitive changes, depression, abuse, and drinking problems. Start low and go slow is the theme for medication assessment. Factors which affect drug absorption, distribution, metabolism and excretion are discussed. A case study and care plan are included.

KEY TERMS

garagenesis	memory recall
developmental tasks	abuse and neglect
cognition	

TEACHING/CLINICAL STRATEGIES

1. Invite a geriatric nurse specialist to discuss the vulnerability and nursing management of critically ill elderly clients which have physical and cognitive changes.

2. Arrange for a pharmacist to lecture about the factors affecting absorption, distribution, metabolism and excretion of medications frequently prescribed for the critically ill elderly.

3. Have students review the medication regimes for their elderly patients to see if there are dose alterations.

4. Have students develop care plans for their elderly clients which identify and address factors associated with advancing age.

Test Questions

1. One of the leading causes of death among older patients is:
   A. diabetes mellitus
   • B. heart disease
   C. renal failure
   D. liver failure

2. A condition that occurs as a result of aging is:
   A. increased resistance to stress
   • B. poor tolerance to extremes of heat and cold
   C. lesser fluctuation in blood ph
   D. increased reaction to external stimuli

3. When an elderly patient is admitted to a critical care unit:
   • A. families are often faced with assuming the role of caring for the patient
   B. families feel they can take a vacation because the nurses will care for the patient
   C. families can make all decisions without problems
   D. families do not have to be concerned about finances because their parents have worked all their lives

4. A plan of care for an elderly patient with hearing loss should include:
   A. shouting at the patient
   B. using a lot of long phrases
   C. standing at least 5 feet from the patient while talking
   • D. remembering not to turn and walk away while talking

5. A major physical change that occurs in the elderly is:
   A. an increase in subcutaneous fat
   B. an increase in the number of sleeping hours
   C. an increased hearing activity

- D. impaired vision

6. A major nursing intervention for an elderly visually impaired patient is to:
   A. approach the patient from the side
   B. get right up to the patient and identify yourself
   - C. allow time for the patient to adapt when moving between dark and light environments
   D. do not use lubricants in the eyes

7. In caring for the elderly patient, it is important to remember that:
   A. intelligence decreases in the elderly
   - B. the elderly are unable to feel the effects of lying in one position too long
   C. usually respond very quickly
   D. maintain strong taste buds

8. A major change in the elderly that occurs with sleep is that:
   A. the time taken to fall asleep is shortened
   - B. less time occurs in REM sleep
   C. total sleep time increases
   D. sleep at night is not interrupted

9. An important consideration about the skin of the elderly is that:
   A. lots of soap should be used on it
   B. sweating increases
   - C. the patient's thermoregulating capabilities are decreased
   D. their skin becomes stronger

10. Cardiovascular changes in the elderly include:
    A. tolerance to quick movements from lying to standing positions
    B. an increase in stroke volume
    - C. loss of arterial elasticity

D. a decrease of pooling of blood in the lower extremities

11. The older patient has:
    A. an increase in expansion of the thorax
    B. increased number of cilia
    C. increased ability to clear secretions
    - D. an increased risk of infection due to possible poor nutrition

12. Changes occurring in the elderly include:
    - A. loss of renal glomeruli
    B. increased peristalsis
    C. increase in bone mass
    D. increase in glucose tolerance

13. Factors that affect drug absorption in the elderly include:
    A. greater lean body mass
    - B. lessened total body fluid
    C. increased glomerular filtration rate
    D. increased creatinine clearance

14. The following is true of the elderly:
    A. metabolism of alcohol does not change
    - B. depression is the leading cause of suicide
    C. short term memory increases
    D. one in 50 elderly people living with their families are abused

15. When medicating an elderly patient, one must remember that:
    - A. the potential for drug interactions increase
    B. drug dosage guidelines are based on studies in the elderly
    C. the elderly do not take over the counter drugs
    D. the elderly have an increased stomach emptying time

CHAPTER **8**

Bioethical Issues in Critical Care

BEHAVIORAL OBJECTIVES

Based on the content in this chapter, the reader
should be able to:

1. Briefly explain the way in which ethics
   assists in reaching answers to moral
   dilemmas.

2. Name the ethical principles most relevant
   to the withholding or withdrawing of
   life-sustaining treatment and the Patient
   Self- Determination Act.

3. Explain the basic difference between the
   two major ethical systems:
   consequentialism and nonconsequential-
   ism.

4. Discuss the terms moral uncertainty,
   moral distress, and moral dilemma.

5. Name the two guidelines that provide the
   nurse with basic directions needed to
   address ethical issues.

OVERVIEW

Chapter 8 describes the process and principles
involved in the systematic study of ethical

dilemmas and includes two case studies which illustrate ethical principles. Content includes definitions of the terms and categories of ethics. The concepts of beneficence, nonmaleficence, autonomy, fidelity and consent are explained. The values and feelings which accompany ethical uncertainties and the reasoning which guides decisions are discussed along with an ethical decision making model.

A section on withholding and withdrawing treatment covers the Patient Self Determination Act, the Hastings Center Guidelines and the ANA Code for Nurses. A DNR situation illustrates the ethical decision making process for withholding treatment.

KEY TERMS

morals	autonomy
ethics	fidelity
bioethics	prima facie
moral uncertainty	obligation
moral dilemma	surrogate
beneficence	

TEACHING/CLINICAL STRATEGIES

1. Invite a nurse ethicist to present a bioethical dilemma and conduct a discussion which illustrates the principles and decision making process in this chapter.

2. Arrange for students to attend an ethics committee in which staff members discuss ethical uncertainties involving their patients.

3. Have students examine the dilemma presented in the following case situation and outline the salient points to consider.

Discuss in class or conference.

4. In conference have students discuss their patient situations which present ethical uncertainties. Help explore situations by using the guiding principles and decision making model in Chapter 8.

THE CASE STUDY

Bill Larson was a 41 year old engineer with testicular cancer. He was admitted to ICU with jaundice, increasing shortness of breath, and excruciating pain from metastasis throughout his body. His pain could only be partially relieved by analgesics. Mr. Larson's status declined rapidly. When Ms. Burke, the primary nurse, spoke with Mr. and Mrs. Larson about the cancer one evening, Mr. Larson told her that the pain was so bad he would welcome death. He requested that she tell Dr. Welch, his oncologist, that he did not want cardiopulmonary resuscitation or "to be put on a machine if anything happened." He was adamant. Mrs. Larson became very angry and said, "No, we want everything done. We're not going to give up now." Then she stormed out of the room.

Late in that shift, Mr. Larson's respiration became increasingly labored. Stat ABGs were very bad, and Ms. Burke knew that Dr. Welch, who was well known for aggressive treatment to the very end, would want to intubate. She spoke with the physician on the telephone and told him of the couple's conflicting desires regarding CPR and ventilators. Dr. Welch replied, "Look, we don't have time for this. He's got to be intubated now, or we'll lose him." Ms. Burke asked, "Why are we intubating him?" she received no response.

As Ms. Burke picked up the phone to notify respiratory therapy of the intubation order, she felt as if she were betraying Bill, but because the situation was urgent and the physician had given an unequivocal order, she saw no other choice.

EXERCISE

What should Ms. Burke do? Using the decision-making model and the ethical principles presented in Chapter 8 in the textbook (*Critical Care Nursing*, 6th Edition), examine this dilemma and outline the salient points to consider.

ANSWERS

Points to Consider

Identification of the Problem. Clinically, the ethical problem involves either (1) violating the patient's wishes and instituting treatment that the wife wants and that the physician has ordered, which will probably prolong the patient's suffering, <u>or</u> (2) affirming the patient's wishes in violation of a direct physician order and the wife's desires, in an emergency situation. At this point, Ms. Burke's options seem limited. She must either act quickly in carrying out the physician's order, or she can choose to not act on the order based on the clearly spoken wishes of Mr. Larson. Both choices have serious consequences for all involved, and one choice seemingly dishonors the principle that justifies the other choice — a true ethical dilemma. The principles of autonomy, beneficence, and fidelity are in deep conflict here.

Relevant Facts and the Ethical Principles Involved. The relevant facts needed to resolve the dilemma include the perspectives of each of those involved. Throughout the night, Bill Larson had been lucid and was **fully aware** (<u>autonomy</u> and

informed consent) of the consequences of foregoing cardiopulmonary resuscitation and intubation. His choice was **clearly articulated** and was based on his belief that, because the pain was so severe at this point and because of his understanding of the prognosis for metastatic cancer, he faced only more pain and debilitation in the future. He felt his **quality of life** (<u>nonmaleficence</u>) was unacceptably poor and that there was no point in prolonging it.

In an ideal situation, decisions that affect more than one person are made with all the individuals participating; **relational discourse (principles of <u>community</u> or <u>solidarity</u>, and <u>fidelity</u>)** provides for sounder decision making because the particular interests, values, and points of view of those involved are expressed and can be arbitrated. If Mrs. Larson had supported her husband's choice to forego CPR, the alternatives available to Ms. Burke might have seemed clearer to her.

At this point, Mrs. Larson does not have a legal or a moral right to make decisions *for* her husband because he has the **capacity** (<u>autonomy</u>) to do so on his own. As his spouse, however, she does have a **moral right to coparticipate** with Mr. Larson in the decision-making process. It is generally assumed that spouses or family members have their loved one's **best interests** (<u>beneficence</u>) at heart. It is at a time when a patient is unable to reason or make a decision known that a spouse (or other surrogate), is commonly looked to make a decision based on his or her knowledge of what the **patient** would have chosen had he or she been able to do so.

Dr. Welch's request for intubation was expected, given the **emergency nature of the situation**. Clearly, he **had not discussed** the use of life-sustaining measures with the Larsons, so his request may have been based on a belief that a "reasonable person" in Mr. Larson's situation would want any and all treatments that would sustain or prolong life. In this case, Dr. Welch may have made an **assumption** that Mr.Larson saw death as the most undesirable consequence and that CPR would provide a **benefit (<u>beneficence</u>)** to him. On the other hand, his order may have been based on an inability to "let the patient go," according to his own values or needs, or on a mistaken interpretation of what the law requires.

Ms. Burke had strong reason to feel uneasy. Developing a **trust relationship (<u>fidelity</u>)** with her patients and enabling them to act on a **self-chosen plan (<u>respect for autonomy</u>)** was of primary importance in her practice and is reinforced as a standard of ethical nursing practice in the *Code for Nurses*. In clearly stating his request to Mrs. Burke, Mr. Larson trusted that she would do what he wanted. Yet Mr. Larson's wife was just as adamant in her demand for life-sustaining measures as he was in his refusal of them.

Responsibilities to the hospital, to the physician, to the patient, to patients' families (**<u>fidelity</u>** in multiple relationships) and to maintaining one's professional integrity (principle of **<u>duties to self</u>**) often cause nurses to have different opinions. The responsibility for Ms. Burke to serve as an **advocate (<u>respect for autonomy and beneficence</u>)** for Mr. Larson's self-expressed wishes is strong and is viewed by the profession as an ethical duty, but the **risks (<u>nonmaleficence and beneficence</u>)** for the nurse are great. If she were to choose not to follow the physician's order, can Ms. Burke expect her supervisor to support such a decision?

<u>Selected Action Alternatives</u>. Refusing to carry out the physician's order would cause problems for Ms. Burke. Would Mr. Larson be justified in expecting her to do so, knowing the personal risks involved? Possibly not. Yet, this action is supported by the ethical principles of respect for autonomy, nonmaleficence, and fidelity. If intubation is not done, Mrs. Larson will have to be dealt with, as it is unlikely that she would see this action as relieving her husband's agony and suffering. She would also need care in dealing with her grief. Dr. Welch would likely be distressed because his orders were not followed. Ms. Burke would be in a position of needing the support of her unit colleagues and the nursing administration, support that might not be forthcoming.

Given the emergency nature of the situation, intubation could be done on a trial basis, thereby stabilizing Mr. Larson's condition. At Ms. Burke's request or insistence, Dr. Welch could then discuss the use of life-sustaining treatments with the couple. (It would of course be necessary for Mr. Larson to still be able to communicate his wishes clearly.) The ventilator could both legally and ethically be withdrawn at that point if that wish were expressed by the patient, although the decision would be an emotionally difficult one.

As another alternative, Ms. Burke could have called Dr. Welch back to explain her concerns more forcefully, in moral rather than clinical terms. Her understanding of the efficacy of CPR on patients with metastatic cancer and her close relationship with Mr. Larson would lend strength to her request to reevaluate the order to intubate.

Other alternatives that Ms. Burke could pursue, though not immediately helpful in this case, would include a request to the institutional ethics committee (IEC) (or to nursing administration if no IEC existed) for the development of a unit or hospital policy on conflicts concerning withholding or withdrawing life-sustaining treatment. In addition, if the hospital had an IEC, or a unit-based ethics committee, or an ethicist-consultant, or a chaplain with a knowledge of ethics, Ms. Burke could have sought assistance from any of those resources.

By definition, ethical dilemmas cannot be resolved either by reducing them to questions of medical or nursing fact by honoring all the principles involved. Different perspectives must be clarified, assumptions must be made known, and the facts and competing values must be weighed against each other. In every situation, the nurse must examine the general ethical principles and professional ethical standards (such as the *Code for Nurses*) as they pertain to the specific features of the individual case. It is not the nurse alone who makes decisions that direct the patient's care; nursing is but one major aspect of health or illness care. But it is the nurse, as a patient advocate, who must see to it that the patient is informed, who gives information where necessary, who facilitates communication, and who ensures that the patient's wishes are known — thus upholding to the best of her or his abilities respect for patient autonomy, professional integrity, and the ethical standards of the nursing profession.

TEST QUESTIONS

1. Choose the most correct answer that describes nursing ethics:
   A. falls under the realm of medical ethics
   B. are based solely on societal values and norms
   - C. are acknowledged as a discipline distinct from medical ethics
   D. include instances where nurses make decisions regarding removal of life support

2. Two major theories of ethical thought include:
   A. utilitarianism and futility
   - B. utilitarianism and deontology
   C. paternalism and futility
   D. none of the above

3. The fundamental principles used in ethical reasoning include:
   A. beneficence
   B. nonmaleficence
   C. autonomy and fidelity
   - D. all of the above

4. Weighing the benefits of an experimental treatment regime to its potentially debilitating side effects is an example of which ethical principle?
   A. autonomy
   - B. beneficence
   C. paternalism
   D. none of the above

5. Informed consent is based on the principle of:
   - A. autonomy
   B. fidelity
   C. nonmaleficence
   D. all of the above

6. Mr. C. is a 60 year old patient with advanced metastatic cancer who is refusing further chemotherapy. His wife is requesting that all possible treatment continue. As his nurse, you would want to be sure that Mr. C.:
   A. has a living will in place
   - B. is fully informed and freely deciding on his withdrawal of chemotherapy
   C. convinces his wife of his wishes
   D. has tried all of his treatment options

7. The 1991 Patient Self Determination Act is intended to assure:
   - A. that hospitalized patients are made aware of their rights to make health care decisions
   B. that surrogate decision makers are available for hospitalized patients
   C. that equal care is provided for all patients
   D. that Ethics Committees exist in hospitals

30

8. A living will:
   A. is required of all hospitalized patients under the Patient Self Determination Act
   B. is the same as a durable power of attorney
   C. is a procedure which allows a person to designate a surrogate to determine treatment decisions
   - D. allows a person to set forth in advance his or her wishes about health care should he or he lose the capacity to make informed decisions

9. Mr. J. is a 36 year old patient with end stage HIV disease. He requests that in the event of a cardiopulmonary arrest he be intubated for one week and if his condition does not improve, the ventilator and endotracheal tube be withdrawn. The nurse should be aware that:

- A. morally, there is no difference between withholding and withdrawing care
   B. Mr. J. should not be allowed to make such constraining decisions
   C. withdrawing care is morally wrong
   D. Mr. J. must have a living will to put forth these wishes

10. Do not resuscitate orders:
   A. are to be ignored when the medical team believes the patient would benefit from the treatment
   B. should be modified based on the differing wishes of the family
   - C. are an example of the patient's fundamental right for selfdetermination
   D. must be made solely by the health care team

CHAPTER 9

Applied Legal Principles

CHAPTER OUTLINE

BEHAVIORAL OBJECTIVES

Based on the content in this chapter, the reader should be able to:

1. Define the four elements of a malpractice suit.

2. Describe the concept of negligence.

3. List three allegations commonly made against nurses.

4. Explain the concept *respondeat superior*.

5. List three possible actions to be taken when there is an unclear medical order, inadequate staffing, or defective equipment.

6. Identify the nurse's responsibilities when there is a do not resuscitate (DNR) order.

7. Summarize five principles that can guide nursing practice.

OVERVIEW

This chapter gives an overview of the four elements of a malpractice suit and describes negligence in critical care. Case examples describe a variety of situations, such as, failures to properly monitor a patient's condition, record observations and notify the physician of abnormalities. Case examples also illustrate the questionable medical order, inadequate staffing and faulty medical equipment. Advance directives are discussed along with orders not to resuscitate, withdrawal of life support and brain death. The summary lists five principles to which the nurse must adhere in order to protect the patient as well as the nurse.

KEY TERMS

negligence	living will
dereliction of duty	health care agent
respondeat superior	power of attorney

TEACHING/CLINICAL STRATEGIES

1. Have students each write statements describing their wishes (advance directives) about life sustaining treatment when they are terminally ill and no longer able to make decisions.

2. In conference or class discuss the circumstances under which CPR may be withheld according to the state's statutes.

3. Arrange for a nurse lawyer to present recent cases involving nurses which demonstrate key points in this chapter.

4. In conference, have students discuss and/or role play how they would respond to the following situations:
   - when there is an unclear medical order;
   - when they are asked to perform something for which they are unprepared;
   - when they are working on a unit which is repeatedly understaffed;
   - when they are asked to move a patient receiving continuous oxygen down the hall without portable oxygen.

TEST QUESTIONS

1. Negligence arises when a nurse:
   A. inflicts injury while giving patient care
   B. causes injury while giving care that other nurses would deem reasonable
   - C. causes injury while giving care that other nurses would deem unreasonable
   D. neglects to follow the established standard of care and no injury results

2. Which of the following areas are often cited in malpractice cases against nurses?
   A. failure to monitor the patient's condition
   B. failure to document observations
   C. failure to notify the physician of abnormalities
   - D. all of the above

3. Hospitals are responsible for the negligent actions of their employees when:
   A. injury results to a patient
   - B. the employee acts within the scope of his or her practice
   C. the employee has no individual malpractice insurance
   D. the employee acts outside the scope of his or her practice

4. The physician writes an order for 12.5 mg Digoxin po q day. The nurse realizes that this dose is 10 times the normal maintenance dose. The nurse should:
   A. give the medication and document his/her concern

B. call the pharmacy for clarification
- C. question the physician who wrote the order
D. withhold the medication and document his/her action

5. In most instances, the nurse who signs as a witness on a consent form is affirming that:
   A. the patient received informed consent
   - B. the patient's signature is not a forgery
   C. the physician's signature is not a forgery
   D. the patient understands the procedure

6. Advance directives include:
   A. living wills
   B. durable power of attorney
   C. attorney in fact
   - D. all of the above

7. Hospitals in compliance with the Patient Self Determination Act must:
   A. assure that all patients have an advance directive
   - B. provide patients with information regarding their right to make decisions about their care
   C. supply the appropriate forms necessary for patients to make advance directives
   D. ask all patients if they would like to create an advance directive

8. When a patient is declared brain dead the health care team should:
   A. continue with life support until the patient's heart stops

- B. discontinue life support unless the patient is to be an organ donor
C. get family permission to terminate life support
D. be aware that declaration of brain death is not legally equated with death.

9. While suctioning an intubated and ventilated patient the nurse notes that the ventilator alarm is malfunctioning. The proper action would be to:
   A. reset the ventilator alarms and monitor it closely for the next few hours
   B. notify the physician of the problem
   - C. remove the ventilator from patient use and report the occurrence to the appropriate person
   D. report the occurrence to the FDA

10. While on duty in a 10 bed ICU, a nurse with no critical care skills/experience is "floated" into the unit to provide patient care. The ICU nurse must be aware that:
    - A. the float nurse should not assume responsibility for aspects of care that he/she is not skilled to give
    B. most hospitals float nurses and policies are in effect to allow this practice
    C. the patient assignment to the float nurse should be the same as for any nurse
    D. inadequate staffing is never an issue in a malpractice lawsuit

CHAPTER 10

Effects of the Critical Care Unit on the Nurse

BEHAVIORAL OBJECTIVES

Based on the content in this chapter, the reader should be able to:

1. Describe the change of focus from initial studies of stress in critical care nurses in the early 1970s to the studies currently being conducted.

2. Identify the self-expectations of critical care nurses that can contribute to burnout.

3. Name the different characteristics of assertive, passive, and aggressive behavior and the reactions of others to those characteristics.

4. Define "coping."

5. Name the personality characteristics described under the coping style of "hardiness."

6. Describe the steps of the quieting reflex.

7. List five changes that can decrease nurses'

stress levels in the critical care unit.

OVERVIEW

Chapter 10 presents information which will help students understand, minimize and cope with job stress. It begins with a review of the literature on stress and its effect on the critical care nurse and then describes the socialization process of the CCU nurse and the stressful factors in CCU's. The personality styles of nurses who are less susceptible to burnout are discussed along with the importance of developing assertive rather than passive or aggressive behaviors. Next, significant stressors reported by CCU nurses are discussed along with interventions to either reduce the stressors or cope with the stress. Group meetings, problem solving and the use of techniques such as the Quieting Reflex are described.

KEY TERMS

assertive

aggressive   hidden agenda

passive   professional
                      distancing
coping

burnout

hardiness

TEACHING/CLINICAL STRATEGIES

1. In conference have students discuss what they find stressful in their critical care experience and share how they currently reduce their stress.

2. In conference have students take about five minutes and list the qualities (using one word descriptions) they expect of themselves as nurses. Have students compare self-expectations. Are they reasonable? Discuss.

3. In conference have students discuss the personality characteristics they think would be ideal for a CCU nurse and their reasons.

TEST QUESTIONS

1. Personality characteristics frequently associated with women include all but the following:
   - • A. achievement oriented behavior
     B. relationship oriented behavior
     C. giving behavior
     D. none of the above

2. A common personality trait frequently associated with nurses is:
     A. assertiveness
     B. aggressiveness
   - • C. selflessness
     D. guilt

3. The feminist movement has caused women and nurses to:
   - • A. become aware of their rights to self fulfillment
     B. experience greater stress in the workplace
     C. feel resentful
     D. all of the above

4. The characteristics of assertive behavior include:
     A. self-esteem
     B. honesty
     C. respect for others
   - • D. all of the above

5. One of the strongest feelings that causes passivity is:
     A. fear
   - • B. guilt
     C. anger
     D. frustration

6. Nurses can learn to have more control in their workplaces by:
     A. being assertive about their beliefs

B. discussing issues instead of repressing feelings
C. learning effective communication techniques
- D. all of the above

7. CCU nurses are found to be different from non-CCU nurses in the following way:
   A. more detached
   B. feel less anxiety
   C. more somatic complaints
   - D. A & B

8. One of the significant factors implicated in job stress is:
   A. conflict with patient's families
   - B. conflict with physicians
   C. the noisy CCU environment

D. poor pay

9. The Quieting Reflex is designed to:
   A. help reduce fatigue
   B. encourage assertiveness
   - C. reduce stress
   D. avoid burnout

10. Nurse managers can foster stress reduction in CCU nurses by:
    A. encouraging group meetings for discussion of feelings
    B. developing appropriate staffing levels
    C. collaborating with psychiatric professionals to facilitate group meetings
    - D. all of the above

CHAPTER **11**

Anatomy and Physiology of the Cardiovascular System

BEHAVIORAL OBJECTIVES

Based on the content in this chapter, the reader should be able to:

1. Briefly describe the characteristics of cardiac muscle cells.

2. Explain the difference between electrical events and mechanical events in the heart.

3. Define *depolarization*.

4. Describe the normal conduction system of the heart.

5. State the formula for calculating cardiac output.

6. Briefly explain the role of the parasympathetic and sympathetic nervous systems in the regulation of heart rate.

7. State the three factors involved in the regulation of stroke volume.

8. Define *preload* and *afterload*.

OVERVIEW

This chapter builds on basic anatomy and physiology and serves as the foundation for understanding pathophysiology and assessment concepts in this cardiovascular unit. It includes details of cardiac micro and macro structure. This paves the way for discussing electrical, mechanical and conduction events in the heart and how these events are reflected on the electrocardiogram.

The physiological principles regulating heart rate, blood pressure and cardiac output are discussed. The aortic and Bainbridge reflexes and the three factors affecting stroke volume (preload, afterload and inotropic myocardial contractility) are described. Coronary and peripheral circulation and their role in tissue perfusion are discussed, as well as blood volume and pressure and the factors which regulate them.

KEY TERMS

action potential	automaticity
resting potential	preload
depolarization	afterload
repolarization	stroke volume
P wave	inotropic
Q wave	cardiac workload
RS wave	Bainbridge reflex
T wave	aortic reflex
PR interval	

TEACHING/CLINICAL STRATEGIES

1. Compare electrical and mechanical events in the heart.

2. Show video/film showing electrical and mechanical events in the heart.

3. Discuss compensatory mechanisms of heart rate, blood pressure, stroke volume and cardiac output and how they may be exhibited in a patient with congestive heart failure.

4. Have students discuss how to assess heart action through observation and by assessing pulses, circulation, skin color and warmth and capillary refill.

TEST QUESTIONS

1. Resting membrane potential is maintained in part by:
   A. active movement of calcium ions into the cell
   B. passive movement of potassium ions out of the cell
   - C. sodium ions being pumped out of the cell
   D. potassium ions being pumped out of the cell

2. The resting potential of the myocardial cell is approximately:
   A. -35mV
   - B. -80mV
   C. +35mV
   D. +80mV

3. The P wave seen on an electrocardiogram (ECG) represents:
   - A. atrial depolarization
   B. atrial repolarization
   C. septal depolarization
   D. ventricular repolarization

4. Which valves are open during diastole:
   A. mitral, aortic
   B. pulmonic, aortic
   C. pulmonic, tricuspid
   - D. mitral, tricuspid

5. A patient's heart rate is 45 beats/minute and regular. The electrical impulse is most likely being initiated by:
   A. the SA node
   B. atrial tissue
   - C. the AV node
   D. the Purkinje fibers

6. Heart rate (HR) will rise in response to:
   A. an increase in arterial blood pressure (BP)
   B. release of acetylcholine

C. stimulation of the parasympathetic nervous system
- D. release of norepinephrine

7. Cardiac output:
   A. will increase in response to decreased ventricular filling
   B. is dependent on body surface area
- C. is normally 4-8 L/minute
   D. is the product of stroke volume and mean arterial pressure

8. If HR = 80 beats/minute, BP = 140/80 mm HG, SV = 100 ml/beat, CO is:
   A. 2 L/min
   B. 4 L/min
   C. 6 L/min
- D. 8 L/min

9. Stroke volume can be increased by:
   A. administration of catecholamines
- B. reducing afterload
   C. reducing preload
   D. increasing systemic vascular resistance

10. Coronary artery perfusion occurs during:
   A. atrial systole
   B. atrial diastole
   C. ventricular systole
- D. ventricular diastole

11. Afterload refers to:
   A. cardiac workload
   B. the amount of stretch placed on cardiac muscle fibers just before systole
- C. the force against which the ventricle must eject blood during systole
   D. the volume of blood in the ventricle at the end of diastole

12. Which of the following is the best indicator of average perfusion pressure:
   A. systolic BP
- B. mean arterial BP
   C. central venous pressure
   D. stroke volume

13. Arterial BP can be reduced in response to:
   A. sympathetic stimulation
- B. stimulation of barorecepotors in the aorta
   C. activation of the renin-angiotensin system
   D. neurally mediated vasoconstriction

14. Decreased entry of calcium into cardiac muscle cells:
   A. increases contractility
   B. causes vasoconstriction
- C. decreases arterial pressure
   D. all of the above

CHAPTER 12

Assessment: Cardiovascular System

BEHAVIORAL OBJECTIVES

Based on the content of this section, the reader should be able to:

1. Discuss four important considerations in preparing a patient for a cardiac examination.

2. Locate the four areas of auscultation on the anterior chest wall.

3. Discuss the mechanisms responsible for the production of the first and second heart sounds and the phases of the cardiac cycle these sounds represent.

4. Discuss the clinical significance of the third and fourth heart sounds and their timing in the cardiac cycle.

5. Describe each type of murmur, its timing in the cardiac cycle, and the area on the chest wall where it is most easily auscultated.

OVERVIEW

Auscultation of the heart builds on concepts mastered in cardiac anatomy and physiology and provides information necessary to conduct a meaningful assessment of heart (rate, rhythm) sounds. Principles underlying the cardiac exam, factors responsible for the production of normal sounds, and the pathophysiology responsible for producing extra sounds, murmurs and friction rubs are discussed.

KEY TERMS

S1, S2, S3, S4

splitting

pericardial friction rub

TEACHING/CLINICAL STUDIES

1. Have students identify the extra heart

sounds diagrammed on the enclosed practice sheet.

2. Have students listen to audiotapes of heart sounds. Students can individually diagram the timing and configuration as they listen.

3. Have students practice locating and auscultating in all four anterior chest areas, first, on each other and then, on each patient assigned for care.

4. Discuss how assessing heart sounds can be important to a patient's well being since it may detect signs of potential cardiac decompensation. Relate to mortality.

5. Discuss how cardiovascular physical examination skills already learned, such as heart rate and rhythm, pulse deficit, Korotkoff sounds, carotid, femoral, posterior tibial and dorsalis pedis pulses, augment auscultation findings.

Section B — Cardiac Enzyme Studies

BEHAVIORAL OBJECTIVES

Based on the content in this section, the reader should be able to:

1. Describe the role of enzyme studies in diagnosing an acute myocardial infarction.

2. Compare and contrast the usefulness of creatine kinase (CK) and lactate dehydrogenase (LDH) isoenzyme studies.

3. List possible etiologies of serum CK and LDH elevations other than acute myocardial infarction—ischemia.

4. Interpret CK and LDH isoenzyme studies when providing patient care.

OVERVIEW

The physiological principles of creatine kinase and lactate dehydrogenase enzymes are discussed, along with their role in detecting cardiac disease and their laboratory values. There is also a focus on the significance and the interpretation of these values in relation to other diagnostic findings.

KEY TERMS

creatine kinase   isoenzyme

lactate
   dehydrogenase

TEACHING/CLINICAL STRATEGIES

1. Discuss how enzymes are useful in diagnosing myocardial injury.

2. Provide a case study or choose a current patient who has had an MI. Review CK and/or LDH isoenzyme studies over a three day period. Discuss normal and abnormal values. Based on the enzymes' response to myocardial infarction, have students relate this patient's enzyme levels to the probable pathophysiological events in the heart. (Refer to the Boxed Display 12-1.)

3. Review this patient's nursing care and discuss how the enzymes levels and myocardial injury are reflected in functional activity level and pain management.

Section C — Cardiovascular Diagnostic Procedures

BEHAVIORAL OBJECTIVES

Based on the content in this section, the reader should be able to:

1. Describe four current techniques used

for diagnostic purposes in cardiology.

2. Outline the patient and family teaching appropriate to prepare the patient for exercise ECG studies.

3. Explain the preparation necessary before cardiac catheterization.

4. Outline the nursing care to be delivered during and after exercise ECG and cardiac catheterization.

5. List potential complications of invasive cardiac studies such as cardiac catheterization.

OVERVIEW

Nine noninvasive and four invasive cardiovascular diagnostic procedures are discussed. The purpose, principles, preparation, procedure, nursing assessment and management are described for each procedure so that nurses can help prepare and support patients and families, and incorporate diagnostic findings into the patient's plan of care.

KEY TERMS

artifact

angiocardiography

doppler
  echocardiography

electrophysiology
  testing

Holter monitor

horizontal plane

infarct imaging

m-mode
  echocardiography

perfusion defect

perfusion imaging

precordial leads

radionuclicide
  imaging

seslamibi

teboroxime

thallium

transesophageal
  echocardiography

two dimensional
  echocardiography

TEACHING/CLINICAL STRATEGIES

1. Have students either role play or actually prepare a patient for an exercise electrocardiography. Discuss student and/or patient responses to the preparation.

2. Have students each observe one of these diagnostic tests, preferably performed on patients for whom they are caring. Ask students how their experiences influenced the ways in which they would prepare patients for the tests.

3. Have each student discuss the test results in relation to the patient's cardiac disease and how the nursing care plan may be altered based on the test findings.

Section D — Electrocardiographic Monitoring

SECTION OUTLINE

Behavioral Objectives

Description

Equipment Features

  Hard-Wire Monitoring Systems

  Telemetry Monitoring Systems

  Monitoring Lead Systems

    Three-Electrode Systems

    Four- and Five-Electrode Systems

    Lead Selection

Procedure

  Electrode Application

  Monitor Observation

Troubleshooting ECG Monitor Problems

Study Questions

BEHAVIORAL OBJECTIVES

Based on the content in this section, the reader should be able to:

1. State the major features of an ECG monitoring system.

2. Discuss the rationale for using the various types of monitoring leads.

3. Describe a method for applying ECG electrodes to achieve an optimal tracing.

4. Identify approaches for troubleshooting ECG monitor problems.

5. List priorities in caring for the patient undergoing ECG monitoring.

OVERVIEW

This section describes principles guiding the three basic components of monitoring systems, the hard wire and telemetry monitoring systems, and the three, four and five lead electrode systems. Electrode application, monitor observation, and troubleshooting monitor problems are also described.

KEY TERMS

oscilloscope

telemetry

negative and positive electrodes

TEACHING/CLINICAL STRATEGIES

1. During clinical experience, observe/demonstrate electrode (re)placement.

2. After (re) placement of the leads briefly discuss the quality of the tracing.

Section E — Dysrhythmias and Conduction Disturbances

BEHAVIORAL OBJECTIVES

Based on the content in this section, the reader should be able to:

1. Define the components used in the evaluation of an ECG tracing.

2. State the criteria for diagnosis of normal sinus rhythm.

3. Identify the ECG criteria used to interpret dysrhythmias commonly encountered in monitored patients.

4. Describe the etiologies, clinical significance, and treatment for each of the dysrhythmias discussed.

5. Discuss the nursing management for those patients exhibiting dysrhythmia disturbances.

OVERVIEW

The waveforms and intervals produced by the ECG and the steps in evaluating a rhythm strip are described. The format for discussing commonly encountered dysrhythmias includes definition, etiology, clinical significance and treatment.

KEY TERMS

PR interval

QRS complex

ST segment

U wave

QT interval

SA Block

Sick Sinus Syndrome

Premature contractions

Paroxysmal supperventricular tachycardia

flutter

fibrillation

multifocal atrial tachycardia

Torsades de Paintes

Bundle Branch Block

TEACHING/CLINICAL STRATEGIES

1. In class or conference evaluate the ECG

patterns of common dysrhythmias using a systematic approach such as the seven steps identified on the transparency (p 62). Have students participate by identifying the dysrhythmia and by discussing the additional signs and symptoms which may be present. Ask if they could determine the presence of this particular dysrhythmia if the patient was not monitored? If so, how?

2. Have students count heart rates, measure waves and intervals and identify the dysrhythmia on practice ECG strips on pages 46 — 51.

3. Have students discuss patients they have cared for (present or past) who have had dysrhythmias. Ask if predisposing factors such as electrolyte imbalance, hypoxemia, pain, fever, etc., (See Care Plan 12-1, item 5).

ANSWERS (SECTION E, QUESTION 2)

1. Ventricular fibrillation
2. Sinus bradycardia with first degree AV block
3. Uniformed ventricular premature beats (VPBs)
4. Premature atrial contractions (PAC's)
5. Premature junctional beat (PJB) - fifth complex
6. Sincus bradycardia
7. Normal sinus rhythm
8. Second degree block - Mobitz II
9. Sinus bradycardia with a sinus arrhythmia
10. Ventricular bigeminy with VPB initiating a run of ventricular tachycardia (VT)
11. Atrial fibrillation with a rapid ventricular response
12. Third degree or complete heart block
13. Atrial flutter
14. Ventricular tachycardia
15. Second degree block - Mobitz I or Weckenbach

Dysrhythmias and Conduction Disturbances

STUDY QUESTIONS

Study each of the following heart tracings, using the questions as a guide. Answer as many of the questions as you can. If you can identify the dysrhythia, write the name above each strip.

1. _____

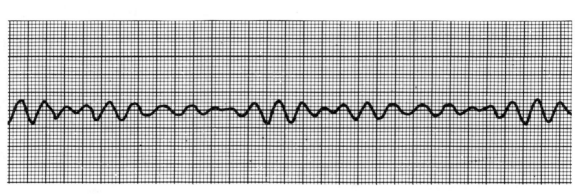

Rate? _____   P — R interval? _____

P wave rate? _____   QRS interval? _____

R wave rate? _____   T wave configuration? _____

2. _____

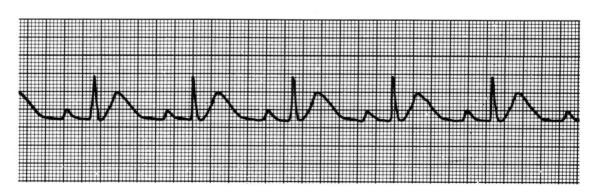

Rate? _____   P — R interval? _____

P wave rate? _____   QRS interval? _____

R wave rate? _____   T wave configuration? _____

3. _____

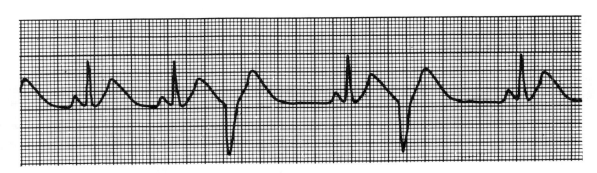

Rate? _____ P — R interval? _____

P wave rate? _____ QRS interval? _____

R wave rate? _____ T wave configuration? _____

4. _____

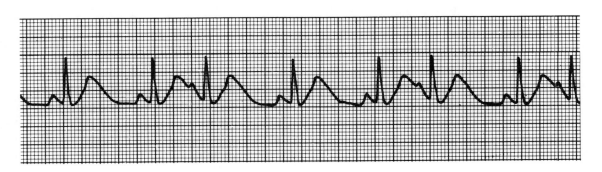

Rate? _____ P — R interval? _____

P wave rate? _____ QRS interval? _____

R wave rate? _____ T wave configuration? _____

5. _____

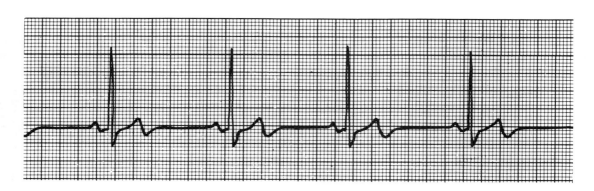

Rate? _____   P — R interval? _____

P wave rate? _____   QRS interval? _____

R wave rate? _____   T wave configuration? _____

6. _____

Rate? _____   P — R interval? _____

P wave rate? _____   QRS interval? _____

R wave rate? _____   T wave configuration? _____

7. _____

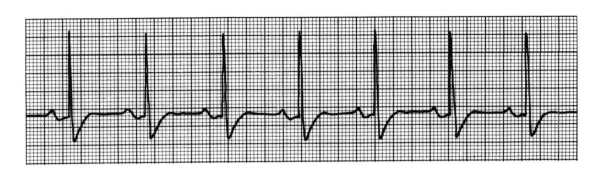

Rate? _____   P — R interval? _____

P wave rate? _____   QRS interval? _____

R wave rate? _____   T wave configuration? _____

8. _____

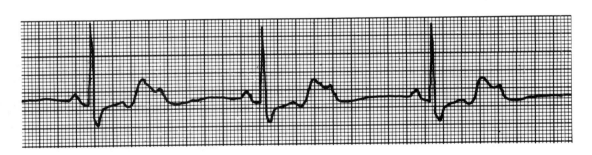

Rate? _____   P — R interval? _____

P wave rate? _____   QRS interval? _____

R wave rate? _____   T wave configuration? _____

9. _____

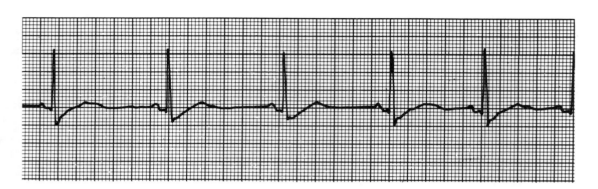

Rate? _____   P — R interval? _____

P wave rate? _____   QRS interval? _____

R wave rate? _____   T wave configuration? _____

10. _____

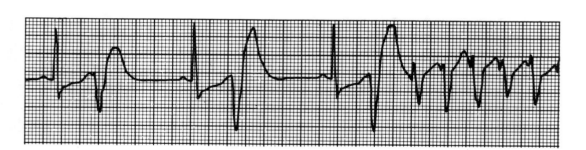

Rate? _____   P — R interval? _____

P wave rate? _____   QRS interval? _____

R wave rate? _____   T wave configuration? _____

11. _____

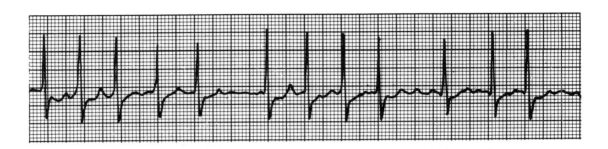

Rate? _____   P — R interval? _____

P wave rate? _____   QRS interval? _____

R wave rate? _____   T wave configuration? _____

12. _____

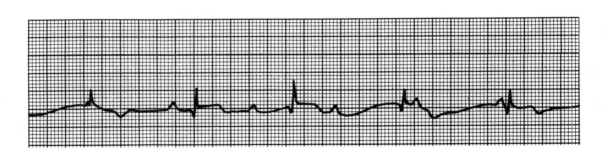

Rate? _____   P — R interval? _____

P wave rate? _____   QRS interval? _____

R wave rate? _____   T wave configuration? _____

Section F — Effects of Serum Electrolyte Abnormalities on the Electrocardiogram

BEHAVIORAL OBJECTIVES

Based on the content of this section, the reader should be able to:

1. Identify common causes of potassium and calcium imbalances in critically ill patients.

2. Describe the ECG changes associated with serum potassium and calcium abnormalities.

OVERVIEW

The effects of too much or too little potassium and calcium on the electrical impulses of the heart are discussed. The focus is to recognize these changes on the ECG before clinical symptoms or hazardous dysrhythmias occur.

KEY TERMS

QT prolongation

TEACHING/CLINICAL STRATEGIES

1. Review the key ECG changes associated with potassium and calcium imbalances. (Refer to Table 12-8 and figures 12 - 45, 46, 48, 49.)

Section G — Hemodynamic Monitoring

SECTION OUTLINE

Behavioral Objectives
Description
Arterial Pressure Monitoring
  Equipment
    Basic Components
    Plumbing System
  Procedure
    Zeroing and Calibrating System
    Arterial Line Insertion
  Interpretation of Results
    Arterial Pressure Waveform
  Management
  Complications
    Infection
    Accidental Blood Loss
    Impaired Circulation to Extremity
Pulmonary Artery Pressure Monitoring Equipment
  Equipment
    Plumbing System
    Swan—Ganz Catheter
  Procedure
    Catheter Insertion
  Interpretation of Results
    Waveforms
      Right Atrial Pressure
      Right Ventricular Pressure
      Pulmonary Artery Pressure
      Pulmonary Capillary Wedge Pressure
      Mixed Venous Oxygen Saturation (S_{vO2})
  Management
Central Venous Pressure Monitoring
  Description
  Procedure
  Interpretation of Results
  Complications
    Infection
    Thrombosis
    Air Embolism
    Line Displacement
Direct Cardiac Output Measurement
  Description

BEHAVIORAL OBJECTIVES

Based on the content in this section, the reader should be able to:

1. Describe the characteristics of a normal systemic arterial, right atrial, right ventricular, pulmonary artery, and pulmonary capillary wedge waveform.

2. Discuss the basic components necessary to monitor pressure invasively.

3. State nursing interventions that ensure accuracy of pressure readings.

4. Discuss the major complications that can occur with an indwelling arterial line and pulmonary artery catheter.

5. Identify nursing interventions to be taken to prevent the above complications.

6. List possible catheter or machine problems that can occur when monitoring pulmonary artery pressures.

7. Describe nursing interventions for troubleshooting equipment problems.

8. Describe the thermodilution method of measuring cardiac output.

OVERVIEW

This comprehensive section discusses the principles, components and skills needed to perform, read and interpret hemodynamic pressures. Pressures include arterial and pulmonary artery pressures, and central venous pressure. Content on direct cardiac output measurement expands on earlier physiological concepts necessary to perform, measure and interpret cardiac output. A focus for each of these procedures is on how this data, along with additional findings, help determine and evaluate therapy.

KEY TERMS

pulmonary capillary wedge wave	Mixed venous oxygen saturation
zero reference point	thermistry circuit
arterial pressure	pulmonary artery diastolic pressure
dicrotic notch	
Swan Ganz catheter	

TEACHING/CLINICAL STRATEGIES

1. Observe at least one type of hemodynamic pressure monitoring either in the clinical area or on video.

2. Have a clinical specialist use patient examples to discuss hemodynamic monitoring focusing not only on the technique but also on how the measurements along with other assessment data contribute to the patient's plan of care.

1. The S2 heart sound is heard best at the:
   A. apex with the diaphragm of the stethoscope
   B. apex with the bell of the stethoscope
   ● C. aortic area with the diaphragm
   D. aortic area with the bell

2. The nurse may auscultate a split S1 in patients with:
   A. congestive heart failure (CHF)
   B. aortic stenosis
   C. a rapid heart rate
   ● D. a right bundle branch block

3. Which of the following will cause a murmur to be heard between S1 and S2:
   ● A. ventricular septal defect
   B. aortic insufficiency
   C. mitral stenosis
   D. pulmonic regurgitation

4. A patient arrives at the hospital complaining of chest pain that began 8 hours ago. Which of the following enzyme studies will be most useful:
   A. serum glutamic- oxaloacetic transaminase (SGOT)
   ● B. creatine kinase (CK)-MB
   C. CK-MM
   D. lactate dehydrogenase (LDH)

5. "Silent ischemia" would most likely be documented by:
   A. 12-lead electrocardiogram (ECG)
   ● B. a holter monitoring
   C. signal-averaged ECG
   D. echocardiography

6. Which of the following signs and symptoms indicate myocardial ischemia during exercise electrocardiography:
   A. ST segment depression of .5mm
   B. increase in heart rate from 80 to 110 beats/minute
   ● C. decrease in systolic blood pressure from 130 to 90mmHg
   D. all of the above

7. The nurse caring for the post-cardiac catheterization patient should:
   A. maintain the patient NPO for at least 6 hours
   B. administer anticoagulants as ordered
   ● C. assess urine output
   D. instruct the patient to ambulate within the first four hours after the procedure

8. Which of the following statements is true about sino-atrial block:
   A. is frequently associated with the respiratory cycle
   B. requires a pacemaker for management
   C. P waves differ in configuration from the sinus P waves
   ● D. one or more P waves are absent

9. Which of the following statements is true about atrial fibrillation:
   A. it has a "sawtooth" appearance on the ECG
   ● B. is frequently present in patients with congestive heart failure (CHF)
   C. cardioversion is the treatment of choice
   D. the atrial rate is between 250-350 beats/minute

10. Your patient with severe cardiac disease is being treated with quinidine and verapamil. He suddenly develops a rapid rhythm characterized by wide QRS complexes of varying amplitude and direction. You:
    ● A. may need to set up for overdrive pacing
    B. prepare to administer lidocaine
    C. defibrillate the patient immediately
    D. prepare to administer additional quinidine

11. Your patient with an acute myocardial infarction has been treated with thrombolytic therapy. His ECG shows a rhythm characterized by regularly occurring wide QRS complexes at a rate of 70 beats/minute. His blood pressure is stable. You:
    A. know that this rhythm may degenerate into ventricular fibrillation

B. prepare to administer a lidocaine infusion
C. prepare the patient for synchronized cardioversion
- D. know that immediate treatment is not necessary

12. Which of the following statements is true about a Mobitz I heart block (Wenckebach):
- A. the PR interval progressively lengthens until a QRS complex is dropped
  B. AV conduction is prolonged, but all impulses are conducted to the ventricles
  C. it may progress rapidly to a third degree heart block
  D. the PR interval is fixed, but non-conducted P waves occur at regular intervals

13. Your patient has CHF and is being treated with digitalis and lasix. You notice his ECG is beginning to show U waves and flattened T waves. Which of the following statements is most likely to be true:
  A. his potassium is elevated
- B. he is at risk of digitalis induced dysrhythmias
  C. his digitalis dose needs to be increased
  D. his calcium level is low

14. Your patient has an auscultated blood pressure (BP) of 130/70 mm HG and a BP of 90/50 mm HG according to his arterial line. Which of the following actions should you take:
  A. do nothing, this is a normal variation
  B. alert the physician, organ perfusion is most likely impaired
  C. reposition the transducer, it is below the tip of the catheter

- D. check the quality of the waveform and correct any damping

15. Left ventricular end-diastolic pressure is best reflected by:
  A. right ventricular diastolic pressure
  B. pulmonary artery (PA) systolic pressure
  C. mean PA pressure
- D. pulmonary capillary wedge pressure (PCWP)

16. A mixed venous oxygen saturation of 45% can be caused by:
  A. a healthy heart responding to exercise
  B. an increase in cardiac output (CO)
- C. a decrease in hemoglobin
  D. the inability of tissues to extract oxygen

17. The PA tracing has spontaneously changed to a PCWP waveform. Which action should the nurse take:
  A. inflate the balloon with 1.5 cc of air
- B. check that the balloon is fully deflated
  C. immediately pull the catheter back to the right atrium
  D. monitor the patient for ventricular ectopy

18. Which of the following values would be characteristic of an acute myocardial infarction:
- A. PCWP = 20 mm HG, CO = 3 L/minute, cardiac index (CI) = 2 L/min/m2
  B. PCWP = 10 mm HG, CO = 7 L/min, CI = 3.5 L/min/m2
  C. PCWP = 18mm HG, CO = 4 L/min, CI = 3 L/min/m2
  D. PCWP = 5 mm HG, CO = 10 L/min, CI = 5 L/min/m2

CHAPTER **13**

Management Modalities: Cardiovascular System

Endocardial Transvenous Pacing

Management

Safety Issues with a Pacemaker

Patient Teaching Regarding a Pacemaker

Complications of Pacing

Failure to Discharge

Failure to Capture Ventricles or Atria

Failure to Sense Spontaneous Beats

Ventricular Irritability

Perforation of Ventricular Wall or Septum

Tamponade

Retrograde Migration of Right Ventricular
Pacing Catheter

Abdominal Twitching or Hiccoughs

Infection and Phlebitis

Migration to Permanent Generator

Malfunction Due to Defibrillation

Nursing Care Plan

StudyQuestions

BEHAVIORAL OBJECTIVE

Based on the content in this section, the reader
should be able to:

1. Describe the functions of each of the three
   pacemaker components: pulse generator,
   leadwire, electrode.

2. Define fixed rate pacing, demand pacing,
   synchronous pacing, and rate-modulated
   pacing.

3. Define AAI, VVI, DVI, DDD and DDDR
   pacing.

4. List the indications for pacemaker therapy.

5. Discuss the potential complications of
   pacemaker therapy and possible
   treatments.

6. Describe the nursing care of a patient with
   both a temporary and permanent

pacemaker.

OVERVIEW

This section is aimed at understanding the
principles of cardiac pacing as a management
modality. Pacemaker components, methods
of pacing, safety issues and the indications for
pacing are discussed. Also covered are
dysrhythmias treated by pacing, key teaching
points, complications, such as perforation of
the septum and tamponade, equipment
problems and infection.

KEY TERMS

asynchronous	tamponade
rate modulated	defibrillation
cardioconverter	migration

TEACHING/CLINICAL STRATEGIES

1. Have students discuss the care of a patient
   who has a pacemaker including key points
   the patient/family need to know by
   discharge.

2. When caring for a patient with a
   pacemaker, discuss how pacing is helping
   the heart maintain rhythm and flow and
   how that is assessed.

Section B — Commonly used Antiarrhythmic Agents and Cardioversion

SECTION OUTLINE

Behavioral Objectives

Pharmacological Agents

Description

Digitalis Preparations

Digoxin
Ouabain
Digitoxin
Digitalis Toxicity
Class I A Antiarrhythmic Agents
Quinidine
Quinidine Toxicity
Procainamide (Pronestyl)
Procainamide Toxicity
Disopyramide
Disopyramide Toxicity
Class I B Antiarrhythmic Agents
Lidocaine
Phenytoin
Tocainide
Mexilitene
Class I C Antiarrhythmic Agents
Encainide and Flecainide
Propafenone
Moricizine
Class II Beta Blocking Agents
Propranolol
Propranolol Toxicity
Acebutolol
Esmolol
Class III Antiarrhythmic Agents
Amiodarone
Bretylium
Sotalol
Class IV Calcium Channel Blockers
Verapamil
Verapamil Toxicity
Diltiazem
Other Antiarrhythmic Agents
Adenosine
Atropine

Assessment and Management
Cardioversion
Description
Procedure
Study Questions

BEHAVIORAL OBJECTIVES

Based on the content in this section, the reader should be able to:

1. Name the most commonly used agents in the treatment of dysrhythmias.

2. State the normal dose and side effects of these common anti arrhythmic agents.

3. Describe the indications and procedure for cardioversion.

OVERVIEW

Content covers the use of drugs and cardioversion in teaching dysrhythmias. Digitalis and several classes of drugs are discussed, including normal doses, desirable and side effects.

KEY TERMS

beta blocking agents   blockers

calcium channel

TEACHING/CLINICAL STRATEGIES

1. Have students care for patients who are receiving one or more of these antiarrhythmic drugs. Discuss the following during clinical conference:

   a) the patient's response to the drug including side effects;

   b) dose considerations for the elderly patient e.g., drug absorption, distribution, metabolism and excretion, (refer to discussion in Chapter 7, The Critically Ill Elderly Patient); and

c) review the dysrhythmias associated with digitalis toxicity and how they may be detected when the patient has a cardiac monitor and when unmonitored.

2. Review the enclosed study questions and ECG strips on commonly used antiarrhythmic drugs.

STUDY QUESTIONS

Commonly Used Antiarrhythic Agents and Cardioversion

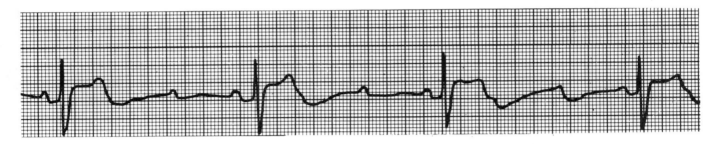

1. A patient with a history of an acute inferior myocardial infarction has an ECG showing the above rhythm. He is also having pain. Which one of the following would be given?

   a. Morphine
   b. Morphine and atropine
   c. O_2
   d. Valium

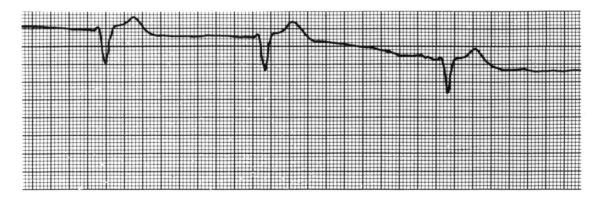

2. A man, age 56, was admitted with severe congestive heart failure. He was given 2.0 mg of digoxin IV with the resulting rhythm. Appropriate R_x now should include *one* of the following:

   a. 0.25 mg digoxin IV
   b. 10 mg KCl IV
   c. Transvenous pacemaker
   d. 1 ampul $CaCl_2$ IV

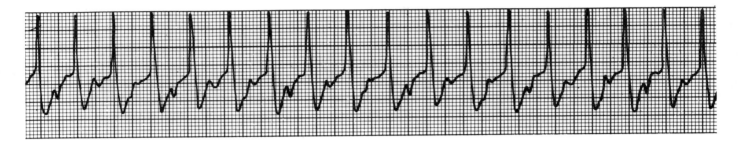

3. The above arrhythmia could result from which *one* of the following?

    a. 100-mg bolus of lidocaine IV
    b. Rapid infusion of isoproterenol (Isuprel)
    c. Excessive sedation with diazepam (Valium)
    d. IV propranolol (Inderal)

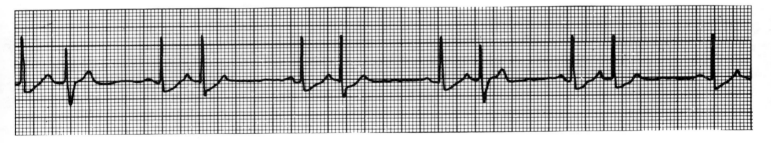

4. The above arrhythmia was observed in a female, age 45. Proper R$_x$ might include *any except one* of the following:

    a. Digoxin
    b. Quinidine
    c. Propranolol (Inderal)
    d. Epinephrine

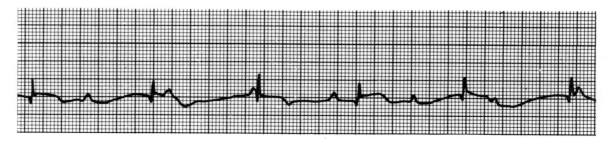

5. Proper R$_x$ of the above arrhythmia might include *all but one* of the following:

   a. IV procainamide (Pronestyl)
   b. Isoproterenol (Isuprel)
   c. Discontinuation of lidocaine drip
   d. Transvenous pacemaker

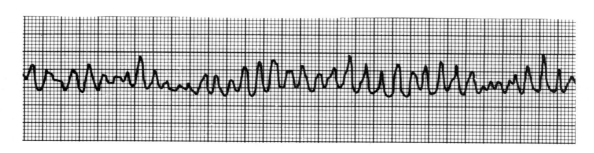

6. If a nurse encounters this rhythm, proper action is to

   a. telephone the operator.
   b. initiate artificial respiration.
   c. check BP.
   d. provide immediate defibrillation.

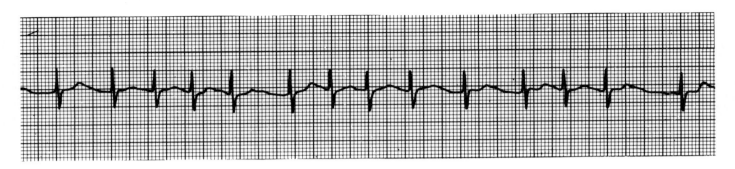

7. A patient on no medication is admitted with the above arrhythmia. The drug of choice is

   a. Lidocaine
   b. Digoxin
   c. Isoproterenol (Isuprel)
   d. IV quinidine

8. If drug R$_x$ of the previous rhythm is unsuccessful, another accepted method of treatment could be:
   a. Pacing
   b. Cardioversion
   c. Heart lung bypass
   d. Mitral commissurotomy

9. This patient was started on procainamide (Pronestyl) 500 mg 6h. Two weeks later she developed signs of Pronestyl toxicity. She might show *all but which one* of the following set of symptoms:
   a. Fainting
   b. Fever, skin rash, and arthritis
   c. positive L.E. cell preps
   d. Yellow vision

10. Ideally, procainimide (Pronestyl) should be administered according to:
    a. Pronestyl blood levels
    b. A "q6h" schedule
    c. Body weight
    d. Size of infarct

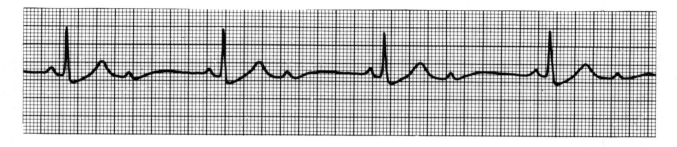

11. This rhythm is important for *all* but *one* of the following reasons:

    a. It may progress to complete heart block.
    b. It should be treated with digitalis.
    c. It will ordinarily respond to isoproterenol (Isuprel).
    d. A transvenous pacemaker should be inserted if the patient has had a myocardial infarction.

12. A patient with a 4 mg/ml drip of lidocaine running rapidly may show which *one* of the following signs:

    a. Fever
    b. diarrhea
    c. Grand mal seizures
    d. Acute gout

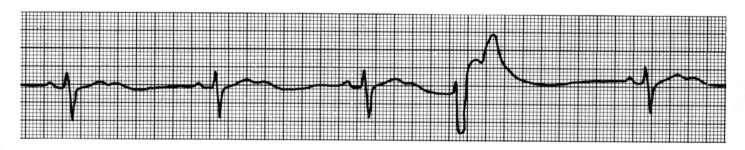

13. A patient with the above rhythm would be treated with which *one* of the following?

    a. Lidocaine
    b. Atropine
    c. Digoxin
    d. Pacemaker

14. Which of the following drugs *decreases* the contractility of the heart muscle?
    a. Digitalis

b. Glucagon
c. Propranolol (Inderal)
d. $CaCl_2$

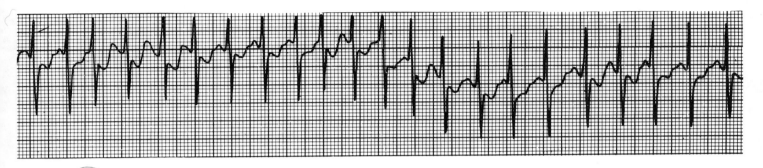

15. Which one of the following is *inappropriate* in treating the above arrhythmia?
    a. Propranolol (Inderal)
    b. Epinepherine
    c. Carotid massage
    d. Digoxin

16. Number the following digitalis preparations in order of rapidity of action and dissipation:
    __ Digoxin
    __ Ouabain
    __ Lanatoside C (Cedilanid)
    __ Digitoxin

17. Which of the following are contraindications for the use of propranolol (Inderal)?
    a. Heart block
    b. Atrial flutter
    c. Congestive heart failure
    d. Chronic lung disease

18. An elderly patient recovering from a myocardial infarction who is on a maintenance dose of quinidine complains of having "blackout" spells. You would suspect:
    a. Postural hypertension
    b. Heart block
    c. Paroxysmal ventricular tachycardia
    d. Small CVAs

19. The nurse's main concern about the digitalized patient who is receiving furosemide (Lasix) is:
    a. Recording I. & O.
    b. Taking CVP readings
    c. Observing for decreasing edema
    d. Observing for arrhythmias due to hypokalemia

20. Which of the following drugs, when used in combination with digoxin, increases the serum level of digoxin by 50% to 70%?
    a. Bretylium
    b. Lidocaine
    c. Tocainide
    d. Verapamil

21. Which of the following antiarrhythmic drugs has a half life of 14 to 52 days, making less frequent dosing a possibility?
    a. Aminodarone
    b. Lorcainide
    c. Propafenone
    d. Encainide

ANSWERS TO STUDY QUESTIONS

1. b. Atropine should be given with a narcotic in the presence of a brady arrhythmia. Atropine will antagonize the tendency of morphine to increase heart block.

2. c. This rhythm strip represents atrial fibrillation with an extremely slow ventricular rate and should be regarded as digitalis toxicity. Transvenous pacemaker is the preferred means of stabilizing the patient with severe heart block. In this case, temporary pacing would be needed until the effects of digitalis toxicity disappeared. Potassium chloride will potentiate the toxic action of digitalis when heart block is present, and potassium is contraindicated in this setting. Calcium chloride also aggravates digitalis toxicity.

3. b. This is a tachyarrhythmia, type unknown, such as can be produced by Isuprel. Lidocaine ordinarily produces no changes in rhythm, and propranolol (Inderal) slows the rate.

4. d. This is atrial bigeminy with some beats aberrantly conducted. Digoxin is the preferred treatment, but quinidine and propranolol (Inderal) are also effective. Epinephrine will increase irritability.

5. a. This patient has complete heart block, and IV Pronestyl would be contraindicated because it could cause ventricular standstill.

6. d. Perform defibrillation if a defibrillator is immediately available. If not immediately available, a blow to the chest may produce enough electrical discharge to defibrillate the heart (5-10 watt sec). Because this rhythm strip represents ventricular fibrillation, maneuvers such as a, b, or c will only delay proper treatment.

7. b. This rhythm is atrial fibrillation with a moderately fast ventricular rate. Isuprel will increase the rate further, lidocaine is ordinarily ineffective for this rhythm, and IV quinidine is contraindicated in *any* patient. Digoxin will slow the ventricular rate, may convert the rhythm to a sinus mechanism, and is the drug of choice.

8. b. Cardioversion. Pacing is ordinarily reserved for abnormally slow rhythms.

9. d. Yellow vision suggests digitalis intoxication due to a toxic effect of this drug on the retina. A, b, c are correct for the following reasons:
   1. Fainting may occur from transient ventricular tachycardia or ventricular fibrillation as a *toxic* effect of Pronestyl.
   2. B and c signify development of lupus-like syndrome occurring fairly common in patients on Pronestyl.

10. a. Blood levels are the most accurate means of monitoring the Pronestyl dose because a high level (8 g/liter) usually correlates with toxicity and a low level (4 g/liter) is often associated with ineffectiveness in controlling the arrhythmia.

11. b. Digitalis (and other drugs such as Pronestyl, quinidine, and Inderal) will increase the degree of heart block present.

12. c. Grand mal seizures are associated with very high levels of licodaine. Usually an AV conduction disturbance would also be present.

13. b. The fourth beat is a ventricular premature contraction (VPB) occurring in a patient with sinus bradycardia. This type of rhythm is commonly seen in the first few hours of infarction. The VPBs usually disappear if the intrinsic heart rate is increased. Atropine will reliably increase the heart rate when sinus bradycardia is present. A pacemaker is usually not necessary unless the rate does not respond to drugs.

14. c. Propranolol (Inderal). The other drugs increase contractility of the heart.

15. b. Epinepherine is appropriate, because it may accelerate the rate further. The rhythm is atrial fibrillation with a rapid ventricular response.

Either digoxin or propranolol (Inderal) is likely to be effective. Carotid massage will slow the rate when atrial fibrillation or atrial flutter is present and often will convert paroxysmal atrial tachycardia to sinus rhythm.

16.
   1. Ouabain
   2. Cedilanid
   3. Digoxin
   4. Digitoxin

17. a,c,d. Heart block may be worsened by Inderal, and standstill may result. *C* is a contraindication because Inderal decreases cardiac contractility and will worsen with congestive heart failure. Inderal may also be contraindicated in chronic lung disease, because it may accentuate bronchospasm. Atrial flutter often responds favorably to Inderal.

18. b,c. Both are toxic manifestations of quinidine. Quinidine produces sudden death in 0.5% of patients who use it chronically, and death is due to arrhythmia.

19. d. Hypokalemia increases the tendency for digitalis toxic rhythms to develop, and potent diuretics such as Lasix and ethacrynic acid, which produce severe potassium loss, should be used with caution in the patient on digitalis. After a dose of Lasix, 20 to 60 mEq/liter of potassium is lost in the urine.

20. d.

21. a.

Section C — Percutaneous Transluminal Coronary Angioplasty and Percutaneous Balloon Valvuloplasty

SECTION OUTLINE

Behavioral Objectives

Description

Percutaneous Transluminal Coronary Angioplasty

History

Physiological Principles

   Mechanisms of Action

Comparisons Between PTCA and CABG

Diagnostic Tests for PTCA and CABG

Patient Selection

Equipment Features

Indications and Contraindications for PTCA

   Indications

   Contraindications

Procedure

Results

Assessment and Management

   Patient Preparation

      Evaluate Lab Tests

      Obtain Informed Consent

      Pre-Op Medications

      Arrange Surgical Standby

   Nursing Management During PTCA

   Nursing Assessment and Management Post-PTCA

Complications

   Angina, Infarction and Vasospasm

   Abrupt Reclosure of Dilated Segment

   Coronary Artery Dissection

   Restenosis

   Other Complications

Nursing Care Plan

The Future of Interventional Cardiology

Percutaneous Balloon Valvuloplasty

History

Pathophysiology of Stenotic Valves

Diagnostic Tests for PBV and Valve Replacement

Equipment Features

Indications and Contraindications for PBV

BEHAVIORAL OBJECTIVES

Based on the content in this section, the reader should be able to:

1. Describe indications and contraindications for percutaneous transluminal coronary angioplasty (PTCA) and percutaneous balloon valvuloplasty (PBV).

2. Discuss interventions for complications associated with PTCA and PBV.

3. List five potential nursing diagnoses and the interventions for each diagnosis in the patient undergoing PTCA

OVERVIEW

This section provides a thorough discussion of these two nonsurgical techniques designed to relieve myocardial ischemia and it's sequela, angina pectoris. Diagnostic tests, the criteria for patient selection, equipment features, procedures, and the results of treatments are included. Patient preparation, assessment and postprocedure management for each technique are discussed and accompanied by a care plan.

KEY TERMS

coaxial   angioplasty

transluminal   stent

recoil

TEACHING/CLINICAL STRATEGIES

Conduct a clinical conference in which post procedure management is discussed, including detecting early signs of complications.

Section D — Intra-aortic Balloon Pump Counterpulsation and Other Ventricular Assist Devices

SECTION OUTLINE

Intra-Aortic Balloon Pump Counterpulsation

Physiological Principles

  Afterload

  Preload

  Contractility

  Heart Rate

Equipment Features

Indications

  Cardiogenic Shock

    Response Patterns

  Postoperative Left Ventricular Failure

  High-Risk Cardiac Surgery

  Septic Shock

  General Surgery for High-Risk Patient

Contraindications

Procedure

  Insertion

  Timing

Interpretation of Results

  Waveform Assessment

BEHAVIORAL OBJECTIVES

Based on the content in this section, the reader should be able to:

1. Describe the physiological effect of intra-aortic balloon pump (IABP) counterpulsation therapy.

2. List indications and contraindications for IABP therapy.

3. Draw and describe the components of an IABP augmented arterial waveform.

4. List five vital assessments the nurse must make during care of the patient receiving IABP therapy.

5. List and describe five potential nursing diagnoses and interventions for each diagnosis.

6. Describe a ventricular assist device that totally supports left ventricular function.

OVERVIEW

These techniques, designed to treat patients' with left ventricular failure, are discussed along with the psychological principles of afterload, preload, contractility and heart rate. Vital concepts include timing of the balloon pump, assessing the waveform, and multiassessment of cardiogenic shock. Complications, troubleshooting and approaches to weaning and balloon pump removal are discussed. There is also information on ventricular assist devices.

KEY TERMS

left ventricular end diastolic pressure	compartment syndrome
intra operative myocardial injury	centrifugal pump
	pulsatile pump

TEACHING/CLINICAL STRATEGIES

1. Have student(s) observe ICU nurses carrying out these treatments, review patient record and share key issues in clinical conference or class.

2. Have a clinical specialist discuss patient preparation, assessment, management and care planning for these treatments during clinical conference or class.

Section E — Autologous Blood Transfusions

SECTION OUTLINE

Behavioral Objectives
Physiological Principles
   Homologous Blood
   Autologous Blood
Equipment Features
Indications/Advantages
   Safety
      Elimination of Disease Transmission
      Elimination of Transfusion Reaction
      Absence of Anticoagulants
   Availability of Blood
   Reduction of Religious Objections
   Cost Effectiveness
Contraindications
Procedure
   Predeposit Phlebotomy (Auto- or Predonation)
   Intraoperative Autotransfusion
   Preoperative Phlebotomy with Hemodilution
   Perioperative and Emergency Autotransfusion
      Postoperative Autotransfusion
      Wound Drainage Reinfusion

   Emergency Autotransfusion
   Continuous Reinfusion Method
   Regional Anticoagulants
Assessment and Management
   General Measures
   Laboratory Studies
   Record Keeping
   Anticoagulation
Complications
   Coagulopathy
Troubleshooting
Nursing Care Plan
Summary
Study Questions

BEHAVIORAL OBJECTIVES

Based on the content in this section, the reader should be able to:

1. Define *autologous blood transfusion*.

2. List five indications for autologous blood transfusion.

3. Explain four methods of autotransfusion.

4. Describe the nursing assessments and interventions necessary for the patient undergoing autotransfusion.

OVERVIEW

This section discusses the principles, equipment, indications and procedures for autologous blood transfusions along with nursing assessment and management.

KEY TERMS

autologous	plasmapheresis
homologous	

71

TEACHING/CLINICAL STRATEGIES

1. Have students discuss the nursing interventions for reducing the risk of hemorrhage, infection and air emboli during reinfusion.

Section F — Cardiopulmonary Resuscitation

SECTION OUTLINE

Behavioral Objectives
Description
Indications/Contraindications
Features of the Resuscitation Team
Assessment of Cardiac Arrest
Procedure for CPR
    Sharp Blow to the Precordium
    Call for Help.
    Achieve Adequate Airway.
    External Cardiac Compression.
    External Countershock.
    Intravenous Infusion.
    Endotracheal Intubation.
    Pharmacological Therapy.
    Countering Cardiac Standstill.
    Ventricular Fibrillation.
    Pericardial Tap.
    Terminating Resuscitation.
Management
    Nursing Care
    Postresuscitative Phase
Complications of Resuscitation
Study Questions

BEHAVIORAL OBJECTIVES

Based on the content in this section, the reader should be able to:

1. Define the terms cardiac arrest, resuscitation, clinical death, and biological death.

2. List symptoms of a cardiac arrest.

3. Describe the role of each member of the resuscitation team.

4. List, in order, the steps of CPR, according to ACLS guidelines.

5. Discuss the first line pharmacologic therapy for cardiac arrest, including indications, dose, route, and side effects.

OVERVIEW

This section of the chapter reviews a 12 step ACLS CPR procedure including the role of the CPR team, pharmacologic therapy and postresuscitation complications and care.

KEY TERMS

cardiac arrest	biological death
clinical death	

TEACHING/CLINICAL STRATEGIES

1. Have students become CPR certified.

2. Have students explore the crash cart. Have a mock code with some students participating in the code and others as observers. In conference have students share observations and reactions and critique performance.

3. If a student observes a resuscitation during clinical experience, arrange attendance at the response team's post code discussion. Have student share both the technical and emotional aspects of the experience during clinical conference.

TEST QUESTIONS

1. A pacemaker is set to discharge whenever the patient's heart rate drops below 50 beats per minute. This is known as:
   A. asynchronous pacing
   - B. demand pacing
   C. synchronous pacing
   D. rate-modulated pacing

2. Which of the following statements applies to VVI mode pacing:
   A. the patient must have an intact AV conduction system
   B. heart rate will change in response to changes in metabolic demands
   - C. the pacemaker senses electrical activity in the ventricle
   D. both atria and ventricles are paced

3. Your patient has a temporary demand pacemaker. You notice an absence of QRS waves after a majority of the pacemaker spikes on his electrocardiogram (ECG).
   A. this is known as failure to sense
   - B. the milliamperage may need to be increased
   C. the pacemaker should be turned off immediately
   D. all of the above

4. Which of the following statements is true regarding digoxin:
   A. it is the drug of choice for sinus tachycardia
   B. it is contraindicated for patients receiving quinidine
   C. dosage should be increased if the patient is hypokalemic
   - D. dosage should be decreased if the patient's serum creatinine level is elevated

5. The drug of choice for treatment of paroxysmal supraventricular tachycardia is:
   - A. verapamil
   B. lidocaine
   C. inderal

D. amiodarone

6. You are caring for a patient with a diagnosis of acute myocardial infarction. She complains of feeling dizzy and you notice that her ECG now shows a sinus bradycardia with a rate of 40 beats per minute. You would prepare to adminster:
   A. lidocaine
   - B. atropine
   C. adenosine
   D. diltiazem

7. During cardioversion your patient's rhythm deteriorates into ventricular fibrillation. Your first action will be to:
   A. administer lidocaine
   B. increase joules to 200 and cardiovert again
   - C. defibrillate the patient
   D. begin CPR

8. Which of the following patients is a candidate for percutaneous transluminal coronary angioplasty (PTCA):
   A. a patient with 90% narrowing of the right coronary artery
   B. a patient with three vessel disease and decreased left ventricular function
   C. a patient with a graft stenosis following coronary artery bypass graft surgery (CABG)
   - D. all of the above

9. Which of the following statements about PTCA is true:
   A. the rate of restenosis is similar to that following CABG
   B. a general anesthetic is required
   - C. complications include angina and infarction
   D. can be used to increase blood flow through stenotic cardiac valves

10. A patient with mitral regurgitation and severe left main coronary artery disease would be a candidate for:
    - A. cardiac surgery

B. PTCA

C. percutaneous balloon valvuloplasty (PBV)

D. intra-aortic balloon pump counterpulsation

11. Intra-aortic balloon pump (IABP) therapy can:

A. reduce cardiac output

B. increase preload

• C. increase blood flow to coronary arteries

D. all of the above

12. Which of the following are contra-indications for the use of IABP:

A. septic shock

• B. aortic insufficiency

C. mitral regurgitation

D. cardiogenic shock

13. During IABP therapy, balloon:

A. deflation enhances coronary perfusion

B. inflation occurs during systole

• C. deflation begins just before the systolic upstroke

D. inflation lasts for 1/3 of the cardiac cycle

14. Complications of autotransfusion include:

A. transmission of hepatitis

B. transfusion reaction

• C. coagulopathy

D. all of the above

15. Which of the following patients is the best candidate for autotransfusion:

• A. a trauma victim with a large hemothorax

B. a Jehova's Witness undergoing surgery for a malignant neoplasm

C. a patient with renal failure undergoing abdominal surgery

D. a patient with a mediastinal infection following cardiac surgery

16. Which drug is most often administered first during a cardiac arrest:

A. sodium bicarbonate

B. bretylium

• C. epinephrine

D. calcium chloride

CHAPTER **14**

Heart Failure

BEHAVIORAL OBJECTIVES

Based on the content in this chapter, the reader should be able to:

1. Describe each of the four reserve mechanisms of the heart.

2. Compare and contrast the etiologies and clinical symptoms of left ventricular failure and right ventricular failure.

3. List the four Killip classifications of heart failure.

4. Explain the vicious cycle of heart failure.

5. Outline the treatment plan for heart failure, including three anticipated pharmacological interventions and three nursing diagnoses.

OVERVIEW

This chapter is appropriate for all students to read during their adult acute care experience.

It discusses the heart's reserve mechanisms, pathophysiology of heart failure and the signs and symptoms of left and right sided failure. Management principles, a case study and care plan are included.

KEY TERMS

dilatation   Laplace relationship

hypertrophy   pressure load

Starling relationship   volume load

TEACHING/CLINICAL STRATEGIES

1. Based on the case study of Mr. White, discuss how the findings described in the first paragraph reflect a failure of the heart's reserve mechanisms and the pathophysiology of cardiac failure. Have students add other signs and symptoms reflective of heart failure.

2. Discuss the implications of the hemodynamic data obtained after intra aortic balloon counterpulsation was initiated.

3. Indicate nursing interventions that are important to Mr. White's physiological and psychological well-being in the next 8 hours.

4. Discuss additional case studies or current patients with heart failure and compare and contrast findings, management, interventions and the patients' response to the plan of care.

TEST QUESTIONS

1. Which of the following compensatory mechanisms helps maintain adequate cardiac output during times of acute stress:
   A. hypertrophy of cardiac muscle
   • B. increase in stroke volume
   C. decrease in venous return
   D. vasodilation

2. Heart failure can result from:
   A. valve malfunction
   B. dysrhythmias
   C. cardiomyopathy
   • D. all of the above

3. Sudden development of a pansystolic murmur, accompanied by onset of acute pulmonary edema and elevated pulmonary artery pressures in a patient with acute myocardial infarction is characteristic of:
   A. pericarditis
   • B. papillary muscle rupture
   C. primary pulmonary hypertension
   D. cardiac tamponade

4. Which of the following is characteristic of left ventricular failure:
   • A. pulmonary capillary wedge pressure (PCWP) = 22 mm HG
   B. right atrial (RA) pressure = 20 mm HG
   C. pulmonary artery pressure (PAP) = 20/10 mm HG
   D. PCWP = 6 mm HG

5. Which of the following signs and symptoms are associated with right ventricular failure:
   • A. enlarged liver, presence of S3
   B. pulmonary vascular congestion, dysrhythmias
   C. decreased breath sounds, orthopnea
   D. decreased cardiac output, acute pulmonary edema

6. The kidneys respond to heart failure by:
   A. excreting potassium and water
   • B. retaining sodium and water
   C. dilating renal vessels
   D. decreasing venous return

7. Cardiogenic shock:
   A. is easily reversed with treatment
   B. is associated with a cardiac index less than 4 L/min/m2

C. is evidenced by a systolic blood pressure less than 80 mm HG
- D. all of the above

8. Which of the following treatments or actions will serve to decrease preload in the patient with left ventricular failure:
   - A. bed rest
   - B. administration of intravenous morphine
   - C. salt and water restriction
   - D. all of the above

9. Which of the following drugs have a vasodilatory action:
   - A. digitalis
   - B. lidocaine
   - C. calcium
   - D. morphine

10. The use of nitroprusside in the treatment of heart failure serves to:
    - A. improve cardiac contractility
    - B. decrease afterload
    - C. increase myocardial oxygen demand
    - D. decrease preload

11. Your patient is receiving a dopamine infusion at 5 micrograms/kg. You would expect to see:
    - A. cool and clammy skin due to vasoconstriction
    - B. a decrease in heart rate and stroke volume
    - C. an increase in urine output
    - D. a decrease in systemic vascular resistance

12. Dobutamine differs from dopamine in that it:
    - A. stimulates only the alpha-adrenergic receptors
    - B. does not have an effect on the kidneys
    - C. results in less vasoconstriction
    - D. causes more pronounced tachycardia

13. Your patient with left ventricular failure develops hepatosplenomegaly and dependent edema. His RA pressure has increased to 24 mm HG and blood pressure is 100/60 mm HG. You suspect:
    - A. cardiogenic shock
    - B. right ventricular failure
    - C. cardiac tamponade
    - D. rupture of the ventricular septum

CHAPTER 15

Acute Myocardial Infarction

BEHAVIORAL OBJECTIVES

Based on the content in this chapter, the reader should be able to:

1. Describe the continuum of pathophysiological events that occur between angina and acute myocardial infarction (MI).

2. List the three major coronary arteries and the structures supplied by their circulation.

3. Describe the pathophysiology and anticipated interventions for cardiogenic shock.

4. Describe the content offered in patient/family education while the recovering MI patient remains in the critical care unit.

5. List and describe four complications of an acute MI.

OVERVIEW

This is a key chapter for students to read

because of the prevalence of MI and because it applies content from earlier chapters. A discussion of coronary circulation helps in understanding infarct location and the implications for heart action. Pain management, drugs to reduce cardiac workload, anticoagulation therapy, diuresis, and thrombolytic therapy are discussed. Hemodynamic pressures and cardiac output measurements are discussed in relation to the location of the infarct and decreased function including cardiogenic shock. Complications include dysrhythmias associated with MI. A case study pulls together diagnosis, assessment and management.

KEY TERMS

collateral circulation	akinetic
atherosclerosis	subendocardial
intimal	infarct
plaque	Weckenbach
nontransmural	unstable angina
infarct	variant angina
dyskinetic	

TEACHING/CLINICAL STRATEGIES

When caring for a patient with an MI, review the record and identify the area of infarction.

1. Locate the portion of injured myocardium on figure 15-1 or 2.

2. Review cardiac enzyme levels and compare with normal values.

3. If hemodynamic pressure and CO are monitored, compare the measurements to normal. Decide what this information tells you about ventricular function.

4. Describe the parameters being monitored.

5. Review episodes of pain, the treatment and the patient's response.

6. What is this patient's level of activity? What methods are reflected in the record for reducing cardiac workload.

7. What is the patient's biggest concern/worry?

8. Discuss some nursing interventions to ease the process of patient transfer out of the CCU. Apply principles from Chapter 2, Psychosocial Concepts and the Patient's Experience with Critical Illness.

TEST QUESTIONS

1. An anterior wall infarction of the left ventricle is most likely associated with a lesion in the:
   A. right coronary artery (RCA)
   - B. left anterior descending artery (LAD)
   C. circumflex artery
   D. collateral vessels

2. Prinzmetal's angina:
   A. is associated with ST segment depression
   B. is characterized by increasingly severe or frequent attacks of angina
   - C. frequently occurs without precipitating factors
   D. is also known as pre-infarction angina

3. The presence of ST elevation and tall T waves indicates:
   - A. new onset transmural infarct
   B. aging transmural infarct
   C. new onset subendocardial infarct
   D. aging subendocardial infarct

4. What electrocardiogram (ECG) changes would you expect to see with anginal pain:
   A. ST elevation
   B. Q waves
   - C. ST depression
   D. T wave inversion

5. Left ventricular function can be measured by:
   A. an ECG

B. vectorcardiography

C. thallium scintigraphy

• D. cardiac angiography

6. Cardiac contractility and workload can be reduced by administration of:

A. morphine

B. nitroglycerin

• C. nifedipine

D. dopamine

7. Which of the following factors would contraindicate the use of beta-adrenergic blockers following an acute myocardial infarction (MI):

A. systolic blood pressure of 100 mm HG

B. premature ventricular contractions (PVC's)

C. tachycardia

• D. second degree AV block

8. Two hours after you began an infusion of tissue plasminogen activator (TPA), your patient develops an accelerated idioventricular rhythm. Blood pressure is 102/60 mm HG. You:

A. turn off the TPA infusion

• B. realize this is probably a reperfusion rhythm and does not require treatment

C. recognize this as a sign of impending cardiogenic shock

D. administer a lidocaine bolus

9. Following an acute MI, Mr. B. is receiving TPA, lidocaine, and nitroglycerin infusions. Currently he is pain free, has a normal sinus rhythm with elevated ST segments and rare PVC's, and a blood pressure of 82/55 mm HG. You:

• A. reduce the nitroglycerin dose

B. administer a p.r.n. dose of morphine

C. administer a bolus of lidocaine

D. obtain an order for nifedipine

10. Mrs. T. has a heart rate of 124 beats/minute and blood pressure of 90/50mm HG following her acute MI. Pulmonary capillary wedge pressure (PCWP) = 6 mm HG; cardiac index (CI) = 1.8 L/min/m2; urine output = 20 cc/hour. She would benefit most from:

A. a dopamine infusion

• B. volume replacement

C. insertion of an intra-aortic balloon pump (IABP)

D. lasix

11. A PCWP of 25 mm HG and CI of 1.5 L/min/m2 is characteristic of:

A. a normal cardiovascular status

B. hypovolemia

C. pulmonary congestion

• D. cardiogenic shock

12. To maintain systemic pressure during cardiogenic shock, which of the following drugs is preferred:

A. dopamine

• B. dobutamine

C. levophed

D. nitroprusside

13. The IABP enhances coronary artery perfusion:

• A. during balloon inflation

B. during balloon deflation

C. during both inflation and deflation

D. during systole

14. Risk of developing a Mobitz II heart block is highest following:

A. posterior infarction

B. lateral infarction

• C. anterior infarction

D. right ventricular infarction

15. Which of the following is true regarding right ventricular infarction:

A. it is commonly associated with a posterior left ventricular infarct

• B. management includes volume support

C. treatment focuses on reduction of preload

D. it is associated with a high incidence of heart block

CHAPTER **16**

Cardiac Surgery and Heart Transplantation

CHAPTER OUTLINE

BEHAVIORAL OBJECTIVES

Based on the content in this chapter, the reader should be able to:

1. Compare and contrast the pathophysiological impact of stenosis and insufficiency in the mitral and aortic valves.

2. Describe the cardiopulmonary bypass process.

3. Describe five key assessment areas of concern in the early postoperative period.

4. Discuss causes, assessments, and interventions for the hypotensive postoperative cardiac surgery patient.

5. Relate the nursing care to the pathophysiological events occurring after cardiac transplantation.

OVERVIEW

The two common conditions requiring cardiac surgery (myocardial revascularization and aortic and mitral valve disease) are discussed along with the procedure of open heart surgery. Content includes the goals of immediate postoperative care: adequate ventilation and oxygenation and hemodynamic stability. Hemodynamic pressures, the type of dysrhythmias and the amount of chest tube drainage to expect early in the postoperative course are also discussed.

Heart transplantation covers the indications, criteria and donor considerations for transplantation. Postoperative care is discussed in relation to the transplanted heart's inability to rapidly change its rate, contractility and output due to denervation. These implications are discussed, as well as, rejection and its treatment with immunosuppressants.

KEY TERMS

chordae

annuloplasty

thrombogenicity

homograft

extracorporeal circulation

cardioplegia

hemodilution

cryoprecipitate

orthotopic transplantation

Panel Reactive Antibody (PRA)

TEACHING/CLINICAL STRATEGIES

1. Arrange clinical experience in a cardiac critical care area and/or step down unit.

2. Consider a class presentation by a clinical specialist from a local cardiac critical care unit to discuss pre- and postoperative nursing interventions for patients having bypass surgery.

3. As part of this class, or in clinical conference, have students problem solve psychological implications and clinical interventions for postoperative findings such as heart rate and rhythm, hemodynamic measurements, respiratory function, chest drainage and pain. Provide a case study, a current patient situation, or Mr. C, the text example.

4. Review postoperative teaching for a cardiac surgery patient. Refer to Box Display 16-1 in text for key points.

5. For preoperative teaching, have students role play:

   a) <u>how</u> they would determine what the patient already knew, wanted to know, and should know and

   b) <u>how</u> they would present the information. Groups of three students can each role play a nurse, a patient and an observer who gives feedback about the interactions.

6. Have students construct a postcardiac surgery teaching plan using the text Nursing Care Plan 16-1 and a hospital patient teaching packet as resources. Have students apply the principles in Chapter 6 Patient and Family Teaching. Have students identify key teaching points in the immediate postoperative period through the first week at home.

7. Arrange for student(s) to observe cardiac surgery.

TEST QUESTIONS

1. An advantage of using the internal mammary artery instead of the saphenous vein for myocardial revascularization is:
   A. it is easier to disect
   B. cardiopulmonary bypass time is decreased
   - C. long term patency is greater
   D. the risk of post operative bleeding is reduced

2. Mitral insufficiency:
   A. is commonly due to congenital anomalies
   - B. is associated with elevated left atrial pressures
   C. leads to right heart failure early in the disease process
   D. frequently causes patients to complain of angina and syncope

3. Narrowing of the valvular orifice between the left atrium and left ventricle is known as:
   A. tricuspid stenosis
   ● B. mitral stenosis
   C. tricuspid insufficiency
   D. mitral insufficiency

4. Which of the following patients is the best candidate for a mechanical valve:
   A. a 25 year old female planning pregnancy within the next 5 years
   B. an 80 year old male with multiple medical problems
   ● C. a 50 year old male with history of chronic atrial fibrillation
   D. a 60 year old poorly compliant female

5. Which of the following protect the heart from ischemia during cardiac surgery:
   A. hypothermia
   B. asystole
   C. the use of a cold cardioplegia solution
   ● D. all of the above

6. Immediately following cardiac surgery, Mr. G's mixed venous oxygen saturation (SVO2) level is 85%. This is partly due to:
   ● A. residual effects of anesthesia
   B. hyperthermia
   C. large amounts of blood lost through mediastinal tubes
   D. the presence of a pleural tube with a large air leak

7. Following mitral valve replacement, Mrs. A has a right atrial pressure (RA) of 2 mm HG; pulmonary capillary wedge pressure (PCWP) = 8 mm HG; cardiac output (CO) = 3 L/minute; blood pressure (BP) = 90/60 mm HG. Urine output is 50 cc/hour and she appears very edematous. She would benefit most from:
   A. an infusion of dopamine
   ● B. administration of colloids
   C. a bolus of normal saline
   D. nitroglycerin

8. Mr. G. had coronary artery bypass graft surgery (CABG). His RA = 6 mm HG; PCWP = 14 mm HG; BP = 200/110 mm HG; CO = 2 L/min; systemic vascular resistance (SVR) = 1400 dynes/sec/cm2. He would benefit most from:
   A. lasix
   B. dobutamine
   ● C. nitroprusside
   D. fluid replacement

9. Which of the following patients is the best candidate for heart transplantation:
   ● A. 65 year old with end stage cardiomyopathy and cardiac induced renal insufficiency
   B. 50 year old with severe coronary artery disease (CAD) and diabetic nephropathy
   C. 45 year old with severe CAD and active peptic ulcer disease
   D. 55 year old with three vessel CAD and mitral regurgitation

10. When orthotopic transplantation is performed:
    A. the recipients entire heart is left in place
    B. the recepients ventricles are left in place
    ● C. two sets of P waves are commonly seen on the electrocardiogram (ECG)
    D. two sets of QRS waves are commonly seen on the ECG

11. A patient's donor heart has developed supraventricular tachycardia. Which of the following will decrease the heart rate:
    A. digitalis
    B. carotid massage
    C. Valsava maneuver
    ● D. verapamil

12. Mr. H. has had a heart transplant. During exercise his heart rate:
    A. will not rise above resting levels
    ● B. will rise slowly and remain elevated for a longer period of time
    C. will rise in response to sympathetic nervous stimulation

D. is likely to drop significantly

13. Acute rejection:
    A. occurs immediately after transplant and results in thrombosis and graft necrosis
    B. occurs 3 months to years following transplantation
  • C. is diagnosed by endomyocardial biopsy
    D. is characterized by angina and decreased exercise tolerance

14. Cyclosporine:
  • A. can cause renal failure and hypertension
    B. is used to reverse established rejection

C. can cause bone marrow suppression
D. all of the above

15. Following heart transplant:
    A. the patient is likely to continue to experience anginal pain
    B. the risk of rejection is highest the first 7 - 10 days
    C. immunosuppressive drugs must be taken for 6 months to one year
  • D. signs and symptoms of infection may be masked

CHAPTER 17

Anatomy and Physiology of the Respiratory System

BEHAVIORAL OBJECTIVES

Based on the content in this chapter, the reader should be able to:

1. Explain the components of total lung capacity.

2. Describe the mechanics of respiration.

3. Define lung compliance

4. Compare and contrast perfect ventilation and perfusion with decreased ventilation and perfusion.

5. Outline the process of gas diffusion through the alveoli and into the blood and tissues.

6. State the importance of oxygen saturation when assessing the effectiveness of respiration.

7. Describe the key features of the oxygen dissociation curve.

8. List two brain stem centers that regulate respiration.

9. Describe the compensatory mechanisms that control respiration.

OVERVIEW

The principles in this chapter serve as a foundation for understanding pathophysiology, assessment, diagnostic tests and management concepts involving the respiratory system. The volume, capacity and dynamic measurements of ventilatory function tests and the four mechanisms of ventilation are described. Physiological concepts for understanding perfusion and transportation of gases are discussed. These include ventilation-perfusion ratios and the oxyhemoglobin dissociation curve. Factors regulating respiration are also discussed.

KEY TERMS

tidal volume (V_T)

inspiratory reserve volume (IRV)

expiratory reserve volume (ERV)

residual volume (RV)

inspiratory capacity (IC)

functional residual capacity (FRC)

vital capacity (VC)

total lung capacity (TLC)

minute volume (V_E)

dead space (V_D)

alveolar ventilation

TEACHING/CLINICAL STRATEGIES

1. Have student(s) observe ventilatory testing, compare results with normal values and review the patient's signs and symptoms which may be attributed to the ventilatory impairment.

2. Take a few minutes in class to have students perform the respiratory movements necessary to measure V_T, ERV, RV, IC and VC.

3. When students care for patients with ventilatory impairment, such as CHF with pulmonary congestion or COPD, discuss the work of breathing, its energy requirements, and nursing interventions to conserve energy.

TEST QUESTIONS

1. The volume of air moved in and out with each normal respiration is called:
   A. inspiratory volume
   - B. tidal volum
   C. residual volume
   D. functional capacity

2. Vital capacity is the sum of:
   - A. tidal volume, inspiratory reserve volume (IRV), expiratory reserve volume (ERV)
   B. tidal volume, residual volume
   C. inspiratory capacity, functional residual capacity
   D. inspiratory reserve volume, expiratory reserve volume, residual volume

3. If a patient's respiratory rate = 12 breaths/minute, tidal volume =500 ml, IRV = 3000 ml, ERV = 1000 ml, minute ventilation is:
   A. 4000 ml
   B. 5000 ml
   - C. 6000 ml
   D. 8000 ml

4. A ventilation to perfusion (VQ) ratio of 1.2 may be seen:
   A. in a healthy adult
   - B. with a pulmonary embolus
   C. with atelectasis
   D. with pulmonary edema

5. Which of the following statements is true regarding pulmonary compliance:
   A. as compliance decreases it becomes easier to expand the lungs for inspiration
   B. increased compliance can be seen in pulmonary fibrosis
   C. compliance is directly influenced by gravity
   - D. more energy will be required for breathing if compliance is reduced

87

6. Dead space:
   A. refers to the tendency of the alveoli to collapse
   B. should not be present in the healthy adult
 • C. consists of the air that is not involved in alveolar gas exchange
   D. is the total lung capacity minus the tidal volume

7. Which of the following is true regarding the pulmonary circulatory system:
   A. in an upright individual more air exchange occurs at the base than at the apex of the lung
   B. pulmonary vascular resistance is significantly higher than systemic vascular resistance
 • C. in an upright position pulmonary vascular resistance is lower at the base than at the apex
   D. hypoxia causes pulmonary vasodilation

8. Which of the following is true regarding oxygen transport:
   A. the majority of oxygen is dissolved in plasma
 • B. hemoglobin is necessary to supply tissues with sufficient oxygen levels
   C. oxygen is bound to carbon dioxide in order to be carried to the tissues
   D. all of the above

9. Which of the following factors will increase the affinity of hemoglobin for oxygen:
   A. fever
   B. acidosis
   C. decreased respiratory rate
 • D. hypocapnia

10. A shift to the right on the oxyhemoglobin dissociation curve:
 • A. causes oxygen to be released more readily to the tissues
   B. can be caused by hypothermia
   C. increases the affinity of hemoglobin for oxygen
   D. causes more oxygen to be picked up by hemoglobin in the lungs

11. Acidosis can cause:
   A. cerebral vasoconstriction
   B. decreased ventilation
 • C. stimulation of chemoreceptors in the medulla
   D. all of the above

12. Carotid bodies and aortic bodies:
   A. increase ventilation in response to hypocapnia
 • B. are stimulated by hypoxia
   C. stimulate the medulla to decrease respiratory rate and depth
   D. are activated in response to cerebral vasodilation

13. Which of the following statements is true regarding the patient with longstanding hypercapnia:
   A. the ability to respond to hypoxia may be decreased or absent
   B. treatment of hypoxia will require higher than normal levels of oxygen
 • C. the carotid and aortic bodies may provide the only stimulus to adjust ventilation
   D. the medulla will be highly sensitive to changes in carbon dioxide levels

CHAPTER **18**

Assessment: Respiratory System

BEHAVIORAL OBJECTIVES

Based on the content in this chapter, the reader

should be able to:

1. List five questions to use when gathering history data.

2. Describe four procedures and possible pertinent findings used in respiratory physical examination.

3. Compare and contrast mixed venous and arterial samples for oxygen, carbon dioxide, pH and oxygen saturation.

4. List the normal values for arterial blood gases.

5. Describe the procedure for obtaining ABGs.

6. Given an example, perform a basic analysis of acid-base interpretation.

OVERVIEW

Because all patients need to be comfortable with their breathing, respiratory assessment is a high priority for nurses caring for critically ill patients. This chapter covers a wide range of respiratory assessment data beginning with significant signs and symptoms and physical examination findings. Diagnostic tests include mixed venous blood sampling, oximetry and arterial blood gases. Measuring PO_2, PCO_2, oxygen saturation and acid base balance are discussed. There is also a procedure for drawing arterial blood gases.

The remainder of the chapter describes physiological principles necessary for understanding and interpreting test results. Content covers respiratory and metabolic acidosis and alkalosis and tissue hypoxemia along with the compensatory mechanisms that help maintain acid base balance and tissue oxygenation. Several examples of ABG values are given along with a nomogram for analyzing the data.

KEY TERMS

ankylosing spondylitis

Marie-Strumpell arthritis

intercostal retraction

vesicular

whispered pectoriloquy

acidemia

alkalemia

acidosis

alkalosis

unspecified anions

anion gap

TEACHING/CLINICAL STRATEGIES

1. Have students listen to audiotapes of lung sounds in self study.

2. Have students listen to chest sounds and assess respiratory signs and symptoms during their CCU experience. In an individual or group conference discuss these feelings and their significance in patient care.

3. Include class content on respiratory and metabolic acidosis/alkalosis, compensation, correction and diagnostic tests.

4. During care of patients requiring ventilation, have students review ABG values (PO_2, PCO_2, Ph, bicarbonate and base excess or deficit) and note patient signs and symptoms. In clinical conference have students discuss these findings and their significance in patient care.

5. Have students answer the study questions on blood gas values for a patient with COPD.

TEST QUESTIONS

1. Which of the following would be the most

reliable indicator of decreased oxygen tension:
A. presence of tactile fremitus
B. cyanosis of the finger tips
- C. cyanosis of the lips
D. deep and rapid respirations

2. Bronchial breath sounds:
A. are heard in the periphery of the lungs
- B. are heard in areas of consolidation
C. are low pitched, without a noticable pause between inspiration and expiration
D. are most often heard in asthma

3. A friction rub:
- A. may be present in pleurisy
B. usually clears after coughing
C. indicates consolidation
D. is characteristic of congenstive heart failure

4. A blood sample for mixed venous oxygen saturation determination should be obtained from the:
A. right atrium
B. superior vena cava
C. femoral vein
- D. pulmonary artery

5. An increase in PCO_2:
A. indicates respiratory alkalosis
- B. can be caused by hypoventilation
C. results in an elevated pH
D. is primarily due to loss of bicarbonate

6. Which of the following indicate metabolic acidosis:
A. low pH, high PCO_2
B. high pH, high HCO_3
- C. low pH, low HCO_3
D. high pH, low PCO_2

7. A blood gas of pH = 7.6, $PCO2$ = 40 mm HG, HCO_3 = 30 mEq/L is most characteristic of a patient with:
- A. a large amount of drainage from his nasogastric tube
B. severe diarrhea

C. diabetic ketoacidosis
D. pneumonia

8. Metabolic acidosis with a normal anion gap can be seen in:
- A. renal tubular acidosis
B. lactic acidosis
C. diabetic ketoacidosis
D. salicylate poisoning

9. A patient's blood gas levels are: pH = 7.2, $PCO2$ = 55 mm HG, $HCO3$ = 24 mEq/L. She has a:
A. metabolic acidosis
B. metabolic alkalosis
- C. respiratory acidosis
D. respiratory alkalosis

10. Compensation for respiratory alkalosis:
A. takes several hours to occur
- B. involves renal excretion of $HCO3$
C. is accomplished by the respiratory system
D. involves acid excretion and base retention

11. Arterial blood gas results include a $PO2$ = 84 mm HG and oxygen saturation ($SaO2$) = 95% on 4 L of oxygen. Mixed venous blood gases reveal a $PO2$ = 30 mmHG and $SvO2$ = 50%. This could be due to:
A. pulmonary edema
B. pulmonary embolus
C. pneumonia
- D. heart failure

12. The patient with severe anemia will have:
A. a low oxygen saturation
B. a low $PO2$
- C. less oxygen delivered to tissues
D. all of the above

13. A patient's admission blood gas is pH = 7.39, $PO2$ = 54 mm HG, $SaO2$ = 87%, $pCO2$ = 62 mm HG, $HCO3$ = 34 mEq/L. Which diagnosis is most likely:
A. acute pulmonary embolus
- B. chronic obstructive pulmonary disease
C. renal failure
D. acute poisoning

14. Which of the following blood gases would be most characteristic of a patient with hypoventilation and tissue hypoxia caused by acute respiratory failure:
    A. pH = 7.2, PCO_2 = 50 mm HG, HCO_3 = 24 mEq
    B. pH = 7.5, PCO_2 = 30 mm HG, HCO_3 = 18 mEq
    C. pH = 7.3, PCO_2 = 50 mm HG, HCO_3 = 30 mEq
  • D. pH = 7.1, PCO_2 = 50 mm HG, HCO_3 = 15 mEq

15. A patient is admitted with dehydration due to severe vomiting. Blood tests show metabolic alkalosis, hypokalemia, hypochloremia. Which of the following treatments would be most beneficial:
  • A. normal saline with potassium
    B. bicarbonate
    C. acetazolamide
    D. sedation

CHAPTER **19**

Management Modalities: Respiratory System

CHAPTER OUTLINE

Bronchial Hygiene
Artificial Airways
Chest Tubes
Pharmacological Agents
Ventilatory Support

Section A — Bronchial Hygiene

SECTION OUTLINE

Behavioral Objectives
Description
Bronchial Hygiene Techniques
  Effective Cough and Deep Breathing
  Chest Physioltherapy
    Chest Percussion
    Vibration
    Postural Drainage
    Special Considerations
  Bronchodilator Aerosol Therapy
  Inhaled Moisture
  Intermittent Positive Pressure Breathing
Study Questions

BEHAVIORAL OBJECTIVES

Based on the content in this section, the reader should be able to:

1. Outline a bronchial hygiene plan of care for a specific patient.

2. List and describe the advantages and disadvantages of intermittent positive pressure breathing (IPPB).

3. Describe advantageous positions for postural drainage of any lung field.

Section B — Artificial Airways

SECTION OUTLINE

Behavioral Objectives
Description
Equipment Features
  Airways
    Oral Pharyngeal
    Nasal Pharyngeal
    Endotracheal Tubes
Suctioning Procedure
Humidification
Study Questions

BEHAVIORAL OBJECTIVES

Based on the content in this section, the reader should be able to:

1. Describe the proper placement of an artificial airway.

2. Explain the rationale for care of an artificial airway.

3. Use proper techniques when suctioning an artificial airway.

Section C — Chest Tubes

SECTION OUTLINE

Behavioral Objectives
Description
Physiological Principles
    Chest Anatomy
    Pleural Pressures
Equipment Features
    Chest Tubes
    Drainage Systems
        One-Bottle System
        Two-Bottle System
        Three-Bottle System
        Disposable Drainage Units
        Emerson Pleural Section Pump
Indications for Chest Tube Placement
Procedure
    Chest Tube Insertion
    Chest Tube Removal
Assessment and Management
    Positioning
    Maintaining System Patency
    Drainage Monitoring
    Water Seal Monitoring
Complications
    Dislodgement of Chest Tube
Study Questions

BEHAVIORAL OBJECTIVES

Based on the content in this section, the reader should be able to:

1. Describe the process by which intrapleural negative pressure is generated.

2. List several indications for chest tube placement.

3. Compare and contrast the one, two, and three-bottle chest tube drainage systems.

4. Discuss the nursing interventions necessary to prevent complications in a patient with a chest tube drainage system.

5. Describe the nursing actions required to maintain chest tube patency.

6. State three potential complications due to chest tube stripping.

Section D — Pharmacological Agents

SECTION OUTLINE

Behavioral Objectives
Description
Bronchodilators
Anticholinergic Drugs
Asthma Prophylactic Drugs
Anti-inflammatory Corticosteroid
Oxygen
Antibiotics
Study Questions

BEHAVIORAL OBJECTIVES

Based on the content in this section, the reader should be able to:

1. Name two specific drugs and their mechanisms of action for each category: bronchodilators and anticholingeric drugs.

2. Describe the rationale for categorizing

oxygen as a drug.

Section E — Ventilatory Support

SECTION OUTLINE

Behavioral Objectives
Description
Physiological Principles
  Effects of Mechanical Ventilation
    Compliance
    Static Pressure
Equipment Features
  Oxygen Delivery Systems
  Manual Resuscitator
  Mechanical Ventilators
    Negative Pressure Ventilator
    Positive Pressure Ventilator
    High Frequency Ventilator
    Today's Generation of Mechanical
    Ventilator
  Ventilator Controls
    FIO_2
    Respiratory Rate
    Tidal Volume
    Peak Flow
    Pressure Limit
    PEEP
    Sensitivity
    Sigh
  Ventilatory Modes
    Assist Mode
    Control Mode
    Assist-Control Mode
    IMV Mode
    Pressure Support Ventilation Mode
    Airway Pressure Release Ventilation
    Mode
    Inverse Ratio Ventilation Mode

Indications for Ventilatory Support
  Respiratory Failure
Procedure
  Standard Settings
    FIO_2
    Respiratory Rate and Tidal Volume
    Peak Flow
    PEEP
    Sensitivity
    Dead Space
    Alarm Systems
  Humidification and Temperature
Assessment and Management of the Ventilated Patient
  Airway Care
  Endotracheal Tube Care
  Tube Cuff Pressures
  Gastrointestinal Care
  Nutritional Support
    Respiratory Muscles
    CNS
    Nutritional Replacement
  Eye Care
  Psychological Care
Complications of Mechanical Support
  Airway Complications
  Endotracheal Tube Problems
  Mechanical Problems
  Barotrauma
  Decreased Cardiac Output
  Positive Water Balance
Weaning from Mechanical Ventilation
  Short-term Weaning
  Procedure
    Methods
      T-Piece
      Intermittent Mandatory Ventilation

BEHAVIORAL OBJECTIVES

Based on the content in this section, the reader should be able to:

1. Define respiratory failure.

2. Identify three potential events affecting different body systems that can lead to respiratory failure.

3. Discuss five indications for mechanical ventilation.

4. Compare and contrast the function of a manual resuscitator bag to a mechanical ventilator.

5. Discuss three different modes of mechanical ventilation.

6. Discuss three different types of mechanical ventilators.

7. Explain the physiological impact of mechanical ventilation.

8. Discuss four nursing interventions necessary for care of a patient on a ventilator.

9. Given a set of ABG values, barometric pressure, water pressure, and target PaO_2, calculate the ventilator FlO_2 setting.

10. Describe potential complications of mechanical ventilators.

11. List three criteria for weaning a patient from a ventilator.

12. Outline five clinical signs that warrant evaluation and possible discontinuation of weaning.

13. Differentiate between short-term and long-term weaning procedures.

14. Discuss four nursing interventions necessary when weaning a patient from a ventilator.

OVERVIEW

Five management modalities are discussed in this chapter, each with it's own section. The purpose, principles, assessment, skills and treatments which comprise bronchial hygiene are discussed in the first section. When bronchial hygiene fails to provide adequate oxygenation and CO_2 removal, an artificial airway and ventilatory support become necessary. The artificial airway section describes the features, principles and placement of oral and nasal pharyngeal airways and endotracheal tubes. Suctioning and humidification are also included.

The last section includes thorough coverage of ventilatory support beginning with the physiological effects of mechanical ventilation. Equipment features include selection of a manual resuscitation bag and descriptions of the types of ventilators and their controls and modes. Ventilatory settings and their indications are described in detail followed by assessment and management aspects of care. Airway care, tube cuff pressures and a multisystem approach to care, including psychological aspects, are covered. Complications due to mechanical ventilation and steps for both short and long term weaning are discussed. A care plan for the mechanically ventilated patent is included.

The remaining two sections include chest tube drainage and pharmacological agents. Chest tube drainage includes the principles, equipment and indications for chest tube placement and removal. The nurses' role in positioning, maintaining tube patency and monitoring drainage is discussed. Pharmacological agents focus on the effects of the following agents on the respiratory system: bronchodilators, cromolyn sodium, corticosteroids, antibiotic and oxygen.

KEY TERMS

multifenestrated

maximum inspiratory pressure (MIV)

static pressure

volume cycled

pressure cycled

high frequency ventilator (HFV)

peak flow

positive and expiratory pressure (PEEP)

intermittent ventilatory mode (IVM)

pressure support ventilation (PSV)

airway pressure release ventilation (ARPV)

inverse ratio ventilation (IRV)

fraction of inspired oxygen (FIO2)

TEACHING/CLINICAL STRATEGIES

1. Have students practice deep breathing, percussing, vibration, and coughing and give feedback to each other about their techniques.

2. Have students make ventilator rounds with a respiratory therapist, noting the ventilator parameters and their significance to patient care.

3. Have a respiratory clinical specialist lecture on patients who are receiving mechanical ventilation including, the indications, the type of airway, type of ventilator and the control settings, measurements to monitor, prevention of complications and other aspects of nursing care. Refer to Nursing Care Plan 19-1, The Mechanically Ventilated Patient.

4. Have students view a video which demonstrates suctioning. (A video is usually available from companies which manufacture suction catheters.)

5. Have students observe or participate in suctioning, airway care, and/or ventilator weaning.

6. Provide a case situation or present a current patient who is being weaned from a ventilator. Discuss nursing interventions which consider physiological and psychological factors including the patient's perceptions, fears and goals about weaning. Refer to Chapter 2, Psychosocial Concepts and the Patient's Experience with Critical Illness and discuss interventions which foster patient coping behaviors, increase the patient's sense of control, and help patients develop self-dialogue messages to increase confidence, optimism and hope. Refer to Figure 2-2 which considers physical and sociopsychological well-being and diagram a consensus view of the patient's readiness for weaning.

TEST QUESTIONS

1. The patient with a left lung abcess should be positioned:
   A. prone
   • B. on the left side
   C. on the right side

D. supine

2. Which of the following is true regarding artificial airways:
   A. an oral pharyngeal airway is necessary to provide high flow oxygen
   B. nasal pharyngeal airways are contraindicated in conscious patients
   • C. an endotracheal tube is usually inserted with the patient supine and the neck hyperextended
   D. an oral pharyngeal airway helps to protect the patient from aspiration

3. Your patient's chest tube just fell out. Your first action is to:
   • A. seal off the insertion site
   B. clamp the chest tube
   C. administer oxygen with a rebreather mask
   D. reinsert the chest tube

4. Pharmacologic therapy for the patient with bacterial pneumonia will include:
   A. theophylline
   B. cromolyn sodium
   C. steroids
   • D. antibiotics

5. Which of the following is true regarding oxygen delivery via nasal cannula:
   • A. oxygen is delivered at flow rates less than the patient's inspiratory volume
   B. gastric distention is a common complication
   C. nasal cannula should not be used if the patient is a mouth breather
   D. the patient receives a constant and precise amount of oxygen

6. Low levels of pressure support :
   A. are frequently used to augment oxygen administration by mask
   B. can decrease cardiac output
   • C. will augment the patient's spontaneous breaths when in the intermittant mandatory ventilation (IMV) mode

D. maintains positive airway pressure when using the assist-control mode of ventilation

7. The patient with decreasing lung compliance should be mechanically ventilated with a:
   A. negative pressure ventilator
   B. pressure cycled ventilator
   C. time cycled ventilator
   • D. volume cycled ventilator

8. Which of the following is true regarding IMV:
   A. the ventilator will deliver a preset tidal volume for every breath the patient initiates
   • B. tidal volume can vary for breaths the patient takes in excess of the preset rate
   C. the patient will be unable to initiate any breaths in excess of the preset rate
   D. this mode is only indicated for unconscious patients

9. The addition of dead space to the mechanical ventilatory system can:
   A. reverse respiratory acidosis
   • B. increase pCO2 levels
   C. reverse hypoxia
   D. eliminate the need for positive end expiratory pressure (PEEP)

10. Your patient's PEEP has just been increased from 10 cm H2O to 12 cm H2O. A sign that the patient is not tolerating this change is:
    A. an increase in cardiac output
    B. hypertension
    C. an increase in functional residual capacity
    • D. a decrease in mixed venous oxygen saturation

11. You are caring for a patient on mechanical ventilation with 10 cm of PEEP. The patient becomes suddenly dyspneic. His trachea is deviated towards the left and breath sounds are absent on the right. You suspect:
    A. atelectasis
    • B. tension pneumothorax
    C. pulmonary edema

D. intubation of right mainstem bronchus

12. Mr. B. is mechanically ventilated at an assist control rate of 18 breaths/minute. He is very agitated and seems to be fighting the ventilator. The alarm is indicating "high pressure". Which of the following actions would be most beneficial:
   A. turn off the alarm until Mr. B. calms down
   B. increase the rate on the ventilator
   C. increase the fraction of inspired oxygen (FIO_2)
   • D. obtain an order for sedation

13. Your patient is breathing at her IMV rate of 16 breaths/minute. Tidal volume is set at 600 cc and $FIO_2 = 40\%$. Arterial blood gases are: pH = 7.5, $PO_2 = 80$ mm HG, $PCO_2 = 28$ mm HG, $HCO_3 = 24$ mEq/L. Which of the following actions would be most likely to improve her blood gases:
   A. change her to an assist-control mode
   • B. decrease her IMV rate
   C. increase her tidal volume
   D. increase her FIO_2

14. The risk of aspiration while on mechanical ventilation can be reduced by:
   A. leaving the endotracheal tube's cuff deflated
   B. administering enteral feedings
   • C. inserting a nasogastric tube
   D. administering prophylactic antacids

15. Development of which of the following signs or symptoms would be cause for termination of weaning from mechanical ventilation:
   • A. respiratory rate of 30 breaths/minute
   B. pH = 7.37, $PCO_2 = 42$ mm HG
   C. drop in systolic blood pressure of 10 mm HG
   D. increase in heart rate of 10 beats/minute

CHAPTER **20**

Common Pulmonary Disorders

BEHAVIORAL OBJECTIVES

Based on the content in this chapter, the reader should be able to:

1. Compare and contrast three etiologies for atelectasis.

2. Outline the signs and symptoms frequently seen with atelectasis.

3. Describe the pathophysiology and anticipated management of pneumonia, bronchospasm, pulmonary emboli, pneumothorax, pleural effusion, and flail chest.

4. Correlate the signs and symptoms of chronic obstructive pulmonary disease (COPD) to the anticipated medical management.

OVERVIEW

Ten common pulmonary disorders are described including atelectasis, pleural effusion, respiratory failure and COPD. A description, clinical manifestations and key management points are included for each disorder. This chapter builds on information presented in earlier chapters and provides an opportunity for readers to apply their knowledge. A case study is included for Mr. Blair who has COPD. Key events, clinical findings and management are described during his hospitalization. A care plan is also included.

KEY TERMS

reabsorption atelectasis	compression atelectasis
passive atelectasis	pulmonary interstitium

TEACHING/CLINICAL STRATEGIES

1. Conduct class which compares and contrasts some of the common pulmonary disorders and their management.

2. In class or conference, using the case study for Tom Blair, have students follow his progress and discuss key findings and nursing interventions.

   a.) Have students discuss possible approaches to helping Mr. Blair wean from the ventilator. Debate the approach described. (Integrate concepts in Chapter 2, Psychosocial Concepts and the Patient's Experience with Critical Illness.)

   b.) Discuss a discharge plan for Mr. Blair which incorporates bronchial hygiene and rehabilitation efforts to conserve energy and increase stamina.

3. Have students respond to the enclosed study questions for a patient with COPD and discuss in class or conference.

CASE STUDY AND QUESTIONS: COPD

Mr. Antonio is a 55-year-old man with emphysema/chronic bronchitis. He is the father of six young children. His wife states that he has been unable to work for the past 2 weeks owing to increasing shortness of breath. In addition, his wife states that his mental alertness has markedly decreased.

Mr. Antonio was diagnosed with emphysema/chronic bronchitis 7 years ago. He worked for 30 years in a sawmill and states he has smoked at least one package of cigarettes per day for 30 years. He has been on a home pulmonary care program without formal home health care follow-up. He was last seen by a doctor 6 months ago. Mr. Antonio is admitted to the hospital.

Lab values (6 months ago):

Chest x-ray:	unchanged; no infiltrates
ABGs:	pH $= 7.35$
	$PO_2 = 56$
	$PCO_2 = 70$
	$HCO_3 = 18$

VS: 18,000
B/P 120/80;
P 100; RR 32;
T 101.8

1. What is the significance of the laboratory values?

2. What additional information would you like to have?

Doctor's orders include:

IPPB with Bronkosol q4h

Steam inhalation

Postural drainage

Vigorous cough

Oxygen at 2 L/min

Patient appears to be oriented to surroundings and events.

16 hours later:

Patient is very lethargic (in checking O_2 flow meter you notice flow is at 6L/min). Breath sounds indicate marked increase in secretions.

3. What action should you take?

24 hours later: *Patient is semicomatose*

ABGs: pH $= 7.26$
$PO_2 = 46$
$PCO_2 = 72$

Nurses report that the patient is unable to cooperate with bronchial hygiene. Deep nasotracheal suction has been attempted but was not able to remove a significant amount of secretions. Rhonchi were heard bilaterally in the upper and lower lobes. Respiratory arrest occurred. Patient was intubated, transferred to the ICU, and ventilated for 16 hours. Antibiotic therapy was initiated. Rigorous bronchial hygiene was performed q1-2 hr. Copious amounts of green-tinged foul-smelling secretions were suctioned from the endotracheal tube.

Chest x-ray: decreased infiltrates; cardiomegaly unchanged

ABGs: oxygen setting at 40%
pH $= 7.35$
$PO_2 = 64$
$PCO_2 = 48$

Patient is oriented and alert.

The endotracheal tube is removed 24 hours later. Rigorous bronchial hygiene is continued. Ambulation is begun. The patient is transferred from the ICU to the ward 24 hours later.

4. Develop a list of information to cover for patient and family education.

ANSWERS

1. The ABGs reveal hypoxemia and acidemia secondary to alveolar hypoventilation and hypercapnia and metabolic acidosis. Respiratory acidosis existed 6 months ago, but the abnormality has increased. Metabolic alkalosis existed 6 months ago and was probably a compensatory mechanism for respiratory acidosis. The elevated WBC indicates infection. The LLL infiltrate points to infection. Cardiomegaly could be secondary to right heart failure (*cor pulmonale*), caused by the patient's lung disease.

2.

   a. What are the normal ABGs at patient's altitude?

   b. Were first and/or second ABGs drawn when patient was receiving supplemental O_2? If so, how much?

   c. What has home pulmonary care consisted of? How frequently has it been done? Does the patient/family understand the purpose of home pulmonary care? Why wasn't home health care involved?

d. What patient education has occurred? How much does the patient/family understand about the diagnosis, causative and irritating factors, and therapeutic modalities?

e. Does the patient know when to call the physician? Does he know where to go for emergency help?

f. Does the family understand the cardinal signs of respiratory distress? Do they know when to call the physician and where to go in case of emergency?

g. Are finances a problem? If so, has a social worker been contacted? Is the patient a candidate for Medicaid or Social Security disability?

h. WBC was 18,000. Would like to have a deferential.

i. Did the patient have a cardiomegaly 6 months ago? Chest x-ray report states: "unchanged." (Unchanged from what?)

j. How significant is shortness of breath (*i.e.*, at rest, performing activities of daily living or following exercise)?

k. What medications does the patient take? What is the medication schedule? Does patient/family understand medications, dosage and side effects?

3. a. Decrease the O_2 flow to 2L/min.

b. Did the patient increase the O_2 flow? Does the patient understand the danger of high flow O_2? This should be a goal of patient/family education.

c. Institute rigorous bronchial hygiene therapy, measures to clear secretions. This has been ordered q4h, but has it been rigorous? Need to increase therapy to q2h. Consider suctioning patient if he is not able to cooperate

and/or generate an effective cough for secretion clearance.

4. The crucial elements of this teaching plan should address multiple areas of education, specifying for each the date basic education occurred, how the patient/family demonstrated knowledge, and problem areas. These essential elements are as follows:

a. Basic airway anatomy

b. Basic disease process of COPD

c. COPD may result in:

1. Continuous productive mucus and secretions above normal

2. Decreased natural cleansing mechanism of lungs

3. Decreased size of air passages

4. Increased susceptibility to lung infections

d. Complications of COPD

e. Irritating factors — can make symptoms worse:

1. Smoking

2. Pollution

3. Extremes of weather

4. Household sprays

5. Dust

6. Animal dander

7. Other (specific to patient)

f. Medications — for each:

1. Name

2. Color

3. Description of shape

4. Reason

5. Frequency

6. Dosage

7. Side effects

g. Bronchial hygiene

1. Compressor nebulizer/IPPB
    i. Use of
    ii. Method of breathing
    iii. Method of cleaning
    iv. Trouble-shooting equipment
2. Steam inhalation
3. Postural drainage/chest percussion
4. Forceful/effective cough

h. Importance of hydration

1. Contraindications
2. Type of fluids

i. Importance of exercise

j. Exercise program

1. How much?
2. How often?

k. Pursed lip breathing

l. Breathing retraining (if indicated/ appropriate)

1. What?
2. How?

m. Indications of pulmonary infection — when to call physician

n. Nutrition

1. Small frequent meals
2. Avoid gas-forming foods

o. Name of your pulmonary doctor

p. Your nurses' names

q. Where to call for any questions or problems related to breathing difficulties

r. Other (specific to patient/family)

TEST QUESTIONS

1. In the presence of atelectasis, normal alveolar ventilation could be blocked by:
    A. mucus
    B. fluid
    C. a space occupying lesion
  • D. any of the above

2. Mr. J. has been on prolonged bed rest following a pelvic fracture. Suddenly he becomes dyspneic and confused. His heart rate = 140 beats/minute, blood pressure = 90/50 mm HG, respirations = 36/minute. His oxygen saturation is dropping rapidly. Which of the following conditions has he most likely developed:
    A. flail chest
  • B. pulmonary embolus
    C. tension pneumothorax
    D. pneumonia

3. Your patient has a diagnosis of emphysema. He develops sudden signs of increasing respiratory distress. Breath sounds and chest movement are decreased on the right side. You suspect he has developed:
    A. a flail chest
  • B. a pneumothorax
    C. an empyema
    D. bronchiectasis

4. Immediate management of a tension pneumothorax consists of:
    A. a lung scan
    B. endotracheal intubation
  • C. needle thoracostomy
    D. aggressive antibiotic therapy

5. A flail chest can cause:
  • A. displacement of the mediastinum toward the unaffected side during inspiration
    B. outward bulging of the affected segment during inspiration
    C. increased intrapleural pressure on the affected side during inspiration
    D. all of the above

6. A pleural effusion can be caused by:
    A. increased colloid osmotic pressure of blood
  • B. increased pressure in the lymphatics

104

C. a tear in the bronchus

D. a decrease in surfactant

7. Purulent sputum is most often seen with :
    A. pulmonary embolus
    B. atelectasis
 • C. pneumonia
    D. pleural effusion

8. Which of the following conditions is associated with pleuritic chest pain:
    A. bronchiectasis
    B. bronchospasm
 • C. pulmonary infarct
    D. asthma

9. Management of a flail chest often includes:
 • A. mechanical ventilation
    B. stabilizing the ribs with a binder
    C. bronchodilators
    D. all of the above

10. A patient is admitted with shortness of breath and wheezing. He had been outside shoveling snow when the episode began. History is negative for cough and smoking. Arterial blood gases reveal a decreased PO_2, oxygen saturation, and PCO_2. PH is elevated. His diagnosis most likely is:
    A. chronic bronchitis
 • B. acute asthma
    C. pneumonia
    D. pleural effusion

11. Which of the following disorders is associated with chronic hypoxemia and chronic hypercapnia:
    A. emphysema
    B. asthma
 • C. chronic bronchitis
    D. all of the above

12. Alveolitis with secondary fibrosis is characteristic of:
 • A. pulmonary vasculitis
    B. empyema
    C. chronic bronchitis
    D. asthma

13. A patient is admitted with a history of chronic bronchitis. Currently he complains of difficulty breathing and a cough productive of copious mucopurulent secretions. His symptoms are the result of:
    A. fibrosis of lung tissue
    B. extensive atelectasis
 • C. widening of the airways
    D. bronchospasm

14. A simple way to manage sleep apnea involves:
    A. waking the patient whenever he becomes apneic
    B. endotracheal intubation
    C. administration of sedatives
 • D. nocturnal administration of oxygen

CHAPTER **21**

Adult Respiratory Distress Syndrome

Chapter Outline

BEHAVIORAL OBJECTIVES

Based on the content of this chapter, the reader should be able to:

1. Relate the assessment findings in ARDS to the pathophysiological process.

2. List the major components of the anticipated medical management.

3. Describe four key nursing diagnoses applicable to the patient with ARDS and outline the nursing interventions for each diagnosis.

OVERVIEW

A very complete discussion of ARDS begins with the wide ranging predisposing events and the pathophysiological changes to the alveolocapillary membrane. ARDS hallmarks of respiratory distress, profound hypoxemia and diffuse bilateral alveolar infiltrates are discussed along with the resulting clinical manifestations and diagnostic findings. Management covers the aspects of mechanical ventilation specific to ARDS. Maintaining respiratory function, daily weighing and hemodynamic monitoring to determine and maintain fluid balance, providing enough nutrients to meet the energy required for the work of breathing, and preventing nosocomial infection are the goals of management. A case study and care plan are included.

KEY TERMS

minute   barotrauma
ventilation(V_e)

TEACHING/CLINICAL STRATEGIES

1. Arrange clinical experience caring for patients receiving mechanical ventilation.

2. In class or conference, discuss the pathophysiology and management of a patient with ARDS.

3. Using the Anita Weiss case study have students discuss the following:

   a) the ventilatory settings for Mrs. Weiss, their physiological effects and expected outcomes on ABG's

   b) the significance of Mrs. Weiss's signs and symptoms, the nursing interventions and expected outcomes.

   c) a plan for weaning Mrs. Weiss from mechanical ventilation which considers her respiratory capability as well as her psychosociological response to her illness (refer to Chapter 2 and Figure 2-2: content on adaption to illness).

   d) indicators of Mrs. Weiss's nutritional status, its possible effect on ventilator weaning and nursing interventions.

TEST QUESTIONS

1. Which pathophysiology is associated with ARDS:
   A. fluid from the left heart backing up into the pulmonary system
   - B. fluid leaking into alveoli due to increased permeability of alveolocapillary membrane

C. shunting due to decreased blood flow through pulmonary capillaries
   D. severe bronchospasm leading to impaired gas exchange

2. Which of the following is indicative of early ARDS:
   A. increased compliance
   B. ventilation-perfusion ratio greater than 0.8
   C. refractory hypoxemia with a high PCO_2
   - D. hypoxemia despite high inspired oxygen fractions (FIO_2)

3. Which of the following signs and symptoms are most characteristic of early ARDS:
   - A. PO_2 below 50 mm HG, low PCO_2, high minute ventilation
   B. PO_2 below 50 mm HG, PCO_2 above 50 mm HG
   C. low PO_2, crackles throughout lung fields, elevated pulmonary capillary wedge pressure (PCWP)
   D. hypoxia, respiratory acidosis, confusion, decreased respirations

4. ARDS can be caused by:
   A. pancreatitis
   B. trauma
   C. disseminated intravascular coagulation
   - D. all of the above

5. ARDS is primarily detected by changes in:
   A. lung scan
   B. physical exam
   - C. arterial blood gases
   D. pulmonary function tests

6. The atelectasis associated with ARDS may be managed or reversed by the use of:
   A. 100% FIO_2 for the first 7-10 days
   B. low tidal volumes
   - C. positive end expiratory pressure (PEEP)
   D. chest tubes

7. The use of PEEP may cause:
   A. increased cardiac output
   - B. development of subcutaneous emphysema
   C. decreased compliance

D. decreased functional residual capacity

8. Which of the following will be increased in ARDS:
A. lung compliance
B. pulmonary capillary wedge pressure (PCWP)
• C. pulmonary vascular resistance
D. oxygen delivery

9. Which of the following should be included in the treatment of every ARDS patient:
A. blood transfusions
B. chest tube placement
• C. nutritional support
D. prophylactic antibiotics

10. Oxygen toxicity can be prevented by:
A. keeping the patient's PO_2 below 80 mm HG
B. using the intermittant mandatory ventilation (IMV)mode instead of assist-control
C. administering a tidal volume (V_T) of 10 - 15 ml/kg body weight
• D. using PEEP in order to decrease the amount of FIO_2 required

11. Mr. W. has ARDS. He has had a negative nitrogen balance and hypoalbuminemia for the past several days. Which of the following may occur:
• A. loss of muscle mass and strength of the diaphragm
B. improved ability to wean from the ventilator
C. difficulty weaning from the ventilator due to high levels of carbon dioxide
D. increased compliance and functional residual capacity

12. You are caring for a patient with ARDS. He is currently ventilated with an FIO_2 of 65%, 15 cm of PEEP, V_T of 1000cc, and rate of 20. He becomes suddenly anxious and agitated. His oxygen saturation (SaO_2) has dropped to 84%, respirations = 32 breaths/minute, breath sounds are diminished over the right upper lobe, and subcutaneous emphysema is present over his upper chest. Treatment of his problem will most likely include:
A. increasing PEEP
• B. insertion of a chest tube
C. decreasing FIO_2
D. administration of a fluid bolus

13. Mrs. Z. has ARDS. She is ventilated with an FIO_2 = 50%, 5 cm of PEEP, V_T = 750cc, rate = 16. Coarse rhonchi are heard over upper airways, her SaO_2 has dropped to 85%, and she is agitated. Which action should the nurse take:
A. increase the PEEP
B. reposition the patient
• C. perform endotracheal suctioning
D. obtain an order for a chest radiograph

14. On an FIO_2 of 80% with 10 cm of PEEP, Mr. T's PO_2 = 45 mm HG, SaO_2 = 75%, cardiac output (CO) = 5 L/minute, blood pressure (BP) = 112/60 mm HG, PCWP = 15 mm HG. His PEEP was increased to 15 cm with the following results: PO_2 = 78 mm HG, SaO_2 = 90%, CO = 3 L/minute, BP = 94/60, PCWP = 18 mm HG. Which of the following would be most beneficial:
• A. dopamine
B. furosemide
C. morphine sulfate
D. steroids

CHAPTER **22**

Anatomy and Physiology of the Renal System

CHAPTER OUTLINE

BEHAVIORAL OBJECTIVES

Based on the content in this chapter, the reader should be able to:

1. Identify the structures comprising the nephron: the glomerulus, proximal tubule, loop of Henle, distal and collecting tubules.

2. Describe the functions of the nephron including glomerular filtration, passive and active transport, tubular secretion, and clearance.

3. Discuss normal fluid pressures in the nephron and how they affect glomerular filtration rate (GFR).

4. Explain the relationship of antidiuretic hormone (ADH), renin, and aldosterone to fluid regulation by the kidneys.

5. Describe the mechanisms by which the kidneys help maintain homeostasis.

OVERVIEW

Renal anatomy and physiology provides a foundation for the renal system chapters which follow. Concepts of renal physiology include filtration, transport, secretion and clearance. Content on the kidney's regulatory functions include a description of ADH, renin and aldosterone and the kidney's role in regulating Ph and electrolytes. These principles can be applied to any patient who is at risk for fluid and electrolyte disruptions.

KEY TERMS

hydrostatic pressure	secretion
osmotic pressure	reabsorption
filtration	active transport

osmosis   diffusion

TEACHING/CLINICAL STRATEGIES

1. Have student apply knowledge of renal anatomy and physiology when caring for patients with renal dysfunction.

2. Have students review their patients' medications and determine their nephrotoxicity and the kidney's role in excretion.

TEST QUESTIONS

1. After leaving the proximal tubule, the filtrate enters:
   A. Bowman's capsule
   - B. the loop of Henle
   C. the distal tubule
   D. the efferent arteriole

2. Glomerular filtration rate (GFR) will increase in response to:
   A. decrease in systemic blood pressure
   B. decrease in plasma hydrostatic pressure
   - C. decrease in filtrate osmotic pressure
   D. vasoconstriction of renal vessels

3. How much filtrate is produced by a normal adult:
   A. 75 ml/minute
   B. 100 ml/minute
   - C. 125 ml/minute
   D. 150 ml/minute

4. Secretion is performed by:
   A. all parts of the nephron
   B. proximal tubule cells
   C. the loop of Henle
   - D. distal tubule cells

5. Reabsorption is accomplished by:
   A. diffusion
   B. osmosis
   C. active transport
   - D. all of the above

6. What happens in the loop of Henle:
   - A. water is reabsorbed
   B. glucose is reabsorbed
   C. urea is secreted
   D. chloride is actively transported out of the filtrate

7. The majority of reabsorption occurs in:
   - A. the proximal tubule
   B. the loop of Henle
   C. the distal tubule
   D. the collecting duct

8. Antidiuretic hormone (ADH) secretion:
   A. is stimulated by a decrease in serum osmolality
   B. causes reabsorption of water and sodium
   C. causes secretion of water and sodium
   - D. causes reabsorption of water

9. Aldosterone:
   A. causes vasoconstriction
   - B. causes reabsorption of water and sodium
   C. converts angiotensin I into angiotensin II
   D. increases serum osmolality

10. The filtrate should not contain:
    A. urea
    B. sodium
    - C. protein
    D. creatinine

11. As the kidneys are compensating for alkalosis, which imbalance may result:
    A. hypernatremia
    B. hyperkalemia
    C. hyponatremia
    - D. hypokalemia

12. Hyperaldosteronism can lead to:
    A. hyponatremia
    - B. metabolic alkalosis
    C. metabolic acidosis
    D. hypochloremia

13. The patient with diabetic ketoacidosis will most likely exhibit:
    A. hypokalemia

- B. hyperkalemia
  C. hyponatremia
  D. hypernatremia

14. If a patient's serum pH is 7.5, sodium will most likely be reabsorbed with:
- A. chloride
  B. bicarbonate
  C. potassium

D. hydrogen

15. A patient has a 3 day history of respiratory acidosis. By now his kidneys are most likely:
  A. reabsorbing sodium with hydrogen
  B. reabsorbing sodium with chloride
- C. secreting hydrogen instead of potassium
  D. secreting potassium instead of hydrogen

CHAPTER 23

Assessment: Renal System

BEHAVIORAL OBJECTIVES

Based on the content in this chapter, the reader

should be able to:

1. Describe the pathophysiology of fluid and electrolyte disorders.

2. Identify manifestations of fluid and electrolyte imbalances.

3. Describe the diagnostic tests used in the evaluation of renal status.

4. Describe the nursing assessment and management of patients with fluid and electrolyte disorders.

5. Formulate a nursing care plan for the patient with hyponatremia.

OVERVIEW

This chapter focuses on the pathophysiological principles, assessment and management of fluid and electrolyte disorders. The principles of solute load and its influence on urinary output in the normal kidney are described and then compared with chronic and acute renal failure. This is followed by a discussion of the fluid balance disorders hypo and hypernatremia and hypo and hypervolemia. Next, history and physical examination, and tests to assess renal function and electrolyte balance are described; and a table summarizes electrolyte abnormalities. Content on assessment and management of sodium and water imbalance integrates and expands on earlier concepts including intake, output and weight. A case study and care plan on the patient with hypothermia are included.

KEY TERMS

solute load

hyponatremia

hypernatremia

hypovolemia

hypervolemia

creatinine clearance

hydrometer

refractometer

osmolality   anion gap

TEACHING/CLINICAL STRATEGIES

1. Conduct class on fluid and electrolyte disorders using this chapter and Chapter 22 as a rereading assignment. Apply this content (especially the assessment and management) to a wide range of patient situations including congestive heart failure, cirrhosis, renal failure and burns.

2. Arrange for nursing rounds which focus on patients experiencing fluid and electrolyte disturbances.

3. Arrange for a clinical specialist to discuss the nursing diagnoses and management of patients with differing medical conditions involving fluid and electrolyte disorders.

TEST QUESTIONS

1. Which of the following will result in hyponatremia:
   A. hyperaldosteronism
   • B. increased secretion of antidiuretic hormone (ADH)
   C. administration of hypertonic tube feedings
   D. severe diarrhea

2. Diabetes insipidus is associated with:
   A. increased secretion of ADH
   B. retention of free water
   • C. loss of free water
   D. hyponatremia

3. The most accurate indicator of renal function is:
   A. serum blood urea nitrogen (BUN)
   B. urine osmolality
   • C. creatinine clearance
   D. specific gravity

4. An elevated BUN and normal serum creatinine can be seen with:
   A. renal disease
   B. liver disease
   C. decreased protein intake
 • D. dehydration

5. Urine specific gravity of a patient with diabetic ketoacidosis will be:
   A. fixed at 1.010
   B. fixed at 1.001
   C. low
 • D. high

6. A low serum osmolality can be caused by:
 • A. hyponatremia
   B. hypokalemia
   C. hyperglycemia
   D. presence of lactic acid in the blood

7. A patient with lactic acidosis will probably also have:
   A. a low anion gap
   B. hyponatremia
 • C. hyperkalemia
   D. hypocalcemia

8. Chronic renal failure is associated with:
   A. hypocalcemia, hypokalemia
 • B. hyperphosphatemia, hypocalcemia
   C. hypophosphatemia, hypermagnesemia
   D. hypomagnesemia, hypercalcemia

9. Mr. B. has lost 3 kg over the last several days. His skin is dry, heart rate and respirations are elevated, blood pressure is low with an orthostatic drop, urine output is 15 cc/hour, and hematocrit is 55%. His signs and symptoms are characteristic of:
   A. hypervolemia
   B. hypokalemia
 • C. hypovolemia
   D. hypercalcemia

10. Which of the following signs and symptoms would a patient with syndrome of inappropriate ADH secretion (SIADH) be most likely to evidence:
    A. paresthesias, tetany, muscle cramps
 • B. headache, confusion, lethargy, convulsions
    C. fatigue, nausea, anorexia, ventricular arrhythmias
    D. bradycardia, respiratory paralysis, dry and sticky oral mucus membranes

11. Mrs. K. has mild congestive heart failure. Her serum sodium = 129 mEq/L. She has pitting edema of the ankles and moist rales are heard in bilateral lung bases. She would benefit most from:
    A. hypertonic saline infusion
    B. administration of 5% dextrose in water (D5W)
    C. vasopressin
 • D. furosemide

12. A patient has a serum phosphate = 2 mg/dl and serum magnesium = 0.8 mEq/L. These imbalances may be due to:
 • A. alcoholism
    B. renal failure
    C. cancer
    D. SIADH

13. Your patient has a diagnosis of acute pancreatitis. She is complaining of abdominal pain, muscle cramps, and parasthesias. She seems irritable and has a positive Chvostek's sign. Which of the following electrolyte imbalances does she most likely have:
    A. hypokalemia
    B. hypernatremia
 • C. hypocalcemia
    D. hypermagnesemia

14. Hyperaldosteronism is associated with:
    A. hyponatremia, hypercalcemia
 • B. hypernatremia, hypokalemia
    C. hyperkalemia, hyperphosphatemia

D. hypocalcemia, hypermagnesemia

15. Mr. T's laboratory studies reveal a sodium = 130 mEq/L; potassium = 6.1 mEq/L; calcium = 7.5 mg/dl; phosphate = 5.0 mg/dl; magnesium = 2.5 mEq/L; creatinine = 4.0 mg/dl; and BUN = 45 mg/dl. His diagnosis

most likely is:
A. congestive heart failure
B. Addison's disease
C. alcoholic liver disease
● D. renal failure

CHAPTER **24**

Management Modalities: Renal System

BEHAVIORAL OBJECTIVES

Based on the content in this chapter, the reader should be able to:

1. List four functions of the artificial kidney system.

2. Describe how the artificial kidney interacts with a dialyzing solution to achieve desired changes in blood components.

3. Describe three variables which should be included in the predialysis assessment.

4. Describe ultrafiltration and the circumstances in which this process is used to correct fluid imbalances.

5. Identify one situation in which a patient could benefit from a continuous renal replacement therapy to achieve fluid balance.

6. List three reasons why a patient might experience hypotension during hemodialysis.

7. Identify one electrolyte whose level is usually corrected during hemodialysis and one electrolyte that is usually restored.

8. Describe the role of oral calcium compounds in correcting hyperphosphatemia.

9. Identify two methods the nurse can use to avoid overheparinization during hemodialysis

10. Describe three technical problems that can occur during hemodialysis.

11. Explain the difference between the AV fistula and polytetrafluorethylene (PTFE) graft.

12. Identify two common sites for insertion of central vein catheters for hemodialysis use.

13. Explain why hemodialysis nurses are sometimes involved in performance of therapies such as hemoperfusion and therapeutic plasma exchange.

14. Describe the psychological needs of the patient receiving hemodialysis therapy for

acute renal failure (ARF) versus the person who is on chronic hemodialysis.

15. Define peritoneal dialysis and two ways in which it differs from hemodialysis.

16. List four essential features of nursing care for the patient receiving peritoneal dialysis.

17. Identify two reasons why peritoneal fluid retention may occur during peritoneal dialysis and two nursing measures to alleviate this problem.

18. State three common signs or symptoms of peritonitis.

19. Identify two reasons why the patient receiving peritoneal dialysis may experience pain during the procedure.

20. Define continuous ambulatory peritoneal dialysis (CAPD) and continuous cyclic peritoneal dialysis (CCPD).

OVERVIEW

Hemo and peritoneal dialysis are thoroughly presented in this chapter. There is a clear description of the features of the artificial dialyzer as well as a proteolyses assessment. Complications during dialysis such as fluid and electrolyte imbalance, infection and bleeding are discussed. Practical information is included about preventing, correcting and managing complications. Ways to troubleshoot problems with equipment, such as dialysate concentration and temperature are explained along with the types and problems associated with accessing circulation.

Peritoneal dialysis is compared with hemodialysis and the equipment, procedure, assessment and management are described. There is emphasis on nursing management including monitoring technical and physiological complications.

KEY TERMS

concentration gradient	ultrafiltration
dialyzer	arterio-venous fistula
dialysate	auto graft
dry weight	continuous renal replacement therapies
ultrafiltration	
sequential	

TEACHING/CLINICAL STRATEGIES

1. Arrange a clinical experience in a dialysis unit which includes observation of the hemodialysis procedure, participation in the pre and ongoing dialysis assessment, and a record review for clinical findings, laboratory values and patient progress.

2. Have students listen to bruits and note the types of vascular access and the kinds of problems patients have had maintaining vascular access. Discuss in postconference.

3. Arrange for students(s) to observe peritoneal dialysis in the hospital and share the nursing process during conference.

4. Consider arranging an experience with CAPD patients during home or office visits to note the nursing assessment and the patient's ability to manage.

5. Have students prepare questions to ask dialysis patients in order to learn about their attitudes, coping mechanisms and ability to carry out their treatment regime. Have students talk with patients about these issues during their dialysis experience.

6. Assign the reading of a nursing research article related to the psychosocial response to illness. The research article in this chapter can be included. Have students share findings and identify interventions they can currently incorporate into their nursing practice.

TEST QUESTIONS

1. Which of the following substances are able to pass through the semipermeable membrane during dialysis:
   A. bacteria
   B. red blood cells
   • C. uric acid
   D. proteins

2. Which of the following is true about dialysate:
   A. it is a sterile solution
   • B. it is made up of water and electrolytes
   C. blood cells are frequently added to dialysate
   D. all of the above

3. Hypotension during dialysis is usually a sign of:
   A. disequilibrium syndrome
   B. anxiety about the procedure
   • C. excessive ultrafiltration
   D. infection

4. Mr. J. will be dialyzed within the next 6 hours. He is scheduled to take 20 mg of propranolol in two hours. In order to prevent hypotension during dialysis he should:
   A. take his medication as scheduled
   B. receive 500 cc of normal saline immediately prior to dialysis
   C. take 40 mg of propranolol at the regularly scheduled time
   • D. omit this dose

5. Mr. G. is undergoing dialysis when he begins to complain of headache, nausea, and twitching. He seems agitated and confused. His problems are most likely related to:
   • A. disequilibrium syndrome
   B. anxiety
   C. excessive ultrafiltration
   D. hyperkalemia

6. Which of the following is true regarding disequilibrium syndrome:
   A. it is indicative of bacterial contamination of the dialysate
   • B. it results from rapid shifts of water and electrolytes between the blood and cerebrospinal fluid
   C. the use of sedatives often precipates the syndrome
   D. it can be prevented by the administration of albumin

7. Your patient has been admitted for dialysis. He has a history of congestive heart failure for which he takes digitalis. He tells you that he has been vomiting the last two days. This patient is at an increased risk of which complication during dialysis:
   A. infection
   B. respiratory arrest
   • C. cardiac arrhythmias
   D. tetany

8. The addition of acetate to the dialysate will:
   A. reverse metabolic alkalosis
   • B. correct metabolic acidosis
   C. relieve muscle cramping
   D. bind phosphorous

9. Bone complications associated with chronic renal failure can be minimized by:
   A. increasing the amount of calcium in the dialysate
   B. adding phosphorous to the dialysate
   C. administration of maalox
   • D. administration of calcium carbonate

10. Magnesium levels in the chronic renal failure patient are controlled by:
- A. dialysis
  B. diet
  C. administration of phosphate binders
  D. administration of milk of magnesia

11. Which of the following is true regarding regional heparinization:
  A. the patient's clotting times will be elevated
- B. protamine is used to neutralize the heparin
  C. it is contraindicated if the patient has uremic pericarditis
  D. all of the above

12. Shortly after her dialysis was begun, Mrs. A's return lines showed clear, cherry red blood. This indicates:
  A. normal functioning of the delivery system
  B. dialysate flow rate is inadequate
- C. hemolysis of blood cells
  D. a leak in the system

13. Which of the following is true regarding peritoneal dialysis:
  A. it utilizes pressure differentials to remove fluid and electrolytes

  B. it takes less time to perform than hemodialysis
  C. it is the treatment of choice for severe drug overdose
- D. the dialysate solution must be sterile

14. During peritoneal dialysis:
  A. the dialysate is pumped into the peritoneal cavity
- B. fluid is drained out by gravity
  C. the effluent is a sterile fluid
  D. the procedure is repeated continuously for about 3-4 hours

15. Your patient is undergoing peritoneal dialysis. After several fluid exchanges you notice that the patient's abdomen is distended and blood pressure is elevated. So far, 6500 cc have been infused and 5500 cc have been drained. Which of the following actions would be most appropriate:
  A. obtain an order for antibiotics
- B. turn the patient from side to side
  C. lower the head of the bed
  D. insert a nasogastric tube

CHAPTER **25**

Acute Renal Failure

BEHAVIORAL OBJECTIVES

Based on the content in this chapter, the reader should be able to:

1. Demonstrate knowledge of the causes of acute renal failure (ARF).

2. Describe urine production during the nonoliguric, oliguric and diuretic stages of ARF.

3. Identify the clinical manifestations of hypoperfusion which can lead the ARF: decreased cardiac output, altered peripheral vascular resistance, and

hypovolemia and hemorrhage.

4. Identify the clinical manifestations of ARF according to these categories: Prerenal, Intrarenal, and Postrenal.

5. Discuss nursing assessment parameters used to identify the alteration in ARF.

6. Develop a nursing care plan for managing the shock and postshock states of ARF.

OVERVIEW

Chapter 25 begins by explaining the categories, causes and pathophysiology of acute renal failure. The assessment section describes the clinical course through the nonoliguric, oliguric and diuretic stages and compares the diagnostic findings for the different categories of renal failure.

The three most common causes of decreased renal perfusion are decreased cardiac output, altered vascular resistance and hypovolemia. Managing each of these is discussed along with interventions to maintain urinary flow. The section on complications focuses on preventing acute tubular necrosis by managing volume replacement, acid-base and electrolyte balance, and nutrition. Drug precautions are explored with five questions to consider along with guidelines for drugs to avoid or to give in reduced dosages. Four care plans, one with an accompanying case study, are included.

KEY TERMS

prerenal	necrosis
intrarenal	azotemia
postrenal	diuresis
acute tubular	

TEACHING/CLINICAL STRATEGIES

1. Arrange for student(s) to care for patients with acute renal failure or at risk due to decreased renal perfusion.

2. In conference have students discuss their patients including the assessment and interventions for managing decreased renal perfusion and preventing ATN. Discuss the patients' medications and their effect on the kidneys.

3. Using the case study for Mrs. Landry and Nursing Care Plan 25-4 (The patient with prerenal azotemia and congestive heart failure), have patients discuss the pathophysiological and management concepts from this chapter and apply them to Mrs. Landry's situation.

4. Have students construct a care plan based on the enclosed case study about Kathy Wilson, a patient with Rhabdomyolisis.

CASE STUDY: KATHY WILSON

Eighteen year old Kathy Wilson has been in a body cast as a result of a car accident. Kathy was celebrating because her cast was going to be removed in 2 days. She reported drinking enough beer to cause her to pass out and fall. She was found several hours later, unconscious and laying on her left arm. The body cast had cut off circulation to the left arm. She was taken to the emergency room by ambulance.

When examined in the emergency room Kathy Wilson was awake, alert and complaining of severe left arm pain. A radial pulse was palpable but the arm was slightly mottled and cool with 1+ edema below the elbow. The left arm was very tender to touch and Ms. Wilson could not move it.

Blood pressure was 120/80, HR 102/min and respirations 30/min. Heart sounds and lung sounds were normal. Initial laboratory data revealed the following:

Serum electrolytes

Na	141 mEq/L	Mg 2 mEq/L
	pH 7.30	CK 780 m/l
K	6.7 mEq/L	Phos 4.5 mg/dl
	$PaCO_2$ 34 torr	
Cl	104 mEq/L	BUN 26 md/dl
	PaO_2 97 torr	
CO_2	7 mmol/L	Hct 46%
	SaO2 98%	
Creat.	2 mg/dl	WBC 18,400mm^3
	HCO_2 20 mEq/L	
Calc.	9 mg/dl	

An IV of NS at 150cc/hr was started and a Foley catheter was inserted.

After 24 hours, Ms. Wilson's arm pain continued and the left radial pulse was audible only by doppler. The arm was cool and edema progressed to 2+. A fasciotomy was done on the left arm to relieve the increased compartment pressures.

Ms. Wilson's urine output decreased and then she became anuric, in spite of lasix and renal dos dopamine. Vital signs were BP 160/100 HR 110 RR 50. She was becoming disoriented. Her weight was up by 3 kg since admission; ausvulation revealed lung crackles and S3 and S4 heart sounds.

Repeat lab values were:

Na	130 mEq/L	Mg 3mEq/L
	Ph 7.30	CK 6400 m/L
K	7.5 mEq/L	Phos 6 mg/dl
	$PaCO_2$ 20 torr	
CL	92 mEq/L	BUN 30 mg/dl
	PaO_2 80 torr	
Co_2	6 mmol/L	Hct 40%
	SaO2 90%	
Creat. 7.2 mg/dl		HCO_3 6 mEq/L

Ca 7 mg/dl

DISCUSSION

It was determined that Kathy Wilson had acute renal failure secondary to Rhabdomyolosis. A subclavian catheter was placed for dialysis. Since her kidneys were no longer working, her Mg, Phos, K, Creatinine and BUN were rising. Ca was falling because of phosphate and magnesium increases. Na and Hct were falling because they were diluted in the increased fluids retained by the patient. The increased fluid retention was causing edema and weight gain. Beginning signs of congestive heart failure were evidenced by crackles and extra heart sounds. Develop a nursing care plan for Kathy Wilson, a patient with Rhabdomyolosis.

TEST QUESTIONS

1. Which of the following can be a prerenal cause of acute renal failure (ARF):
   - A. renal artery stenosis
   - B. hypercalcemia
   - C. diabetes mellitus
   - D. kidney stones

2. An obstruction of urine flow between the collection ducts and the external uretheral orifice:
   - A. can not cause renal failure
   - B. is a prerenal cause of ARF
   - C. is an intrarenal cause of ARF
   - D. is a postrenal cause of ARF

3. In ARF due to prolonged hypotension you would expect to see:
   - A. a large amount of casts present in the urine
   - B. a low urine sodium concentration
   - C. urine specific gravity similar to that of plasma
   - D. nonoliguric renal failure

4. Your patient has ARF due to a bilateral ureteral obstruction. You would expect to see a decrease in:
   A. blood urea nitrogen (BUN)
   B. serum creatinine
 • C. urine sodium
   D. urine specific gravity

5. Which of the following patients is most likely to develop a nonoliguric renal failure:
   A. the patient with severe congestive heart failure and a decreased cardiac output
 • B. the patient with an infection receiving gentamycin
   C. the trauma patient with a severe hemorrhage
   D. the patient with malignant hypertension

6. A common complication during the oliguric phase of ARF is:
   A. hyponatremia
   B. dysrythmias due to hypokalemia
 • C. pulmonary edema
   D. metabolic alkalosis

7. Mr. R.'s laboratory studies reveal urine sodium = 35 mEq/L; urine specific gravity = 1.010; urine osmolality = 280 mOsm/L. His renal failure could be caused by:
   A. diabetes mellitus
   B. renal artery stenosis
   C. prolonged hypovolemia
   D. acute pancreatitis

8. Mannitol can be used to:
   A. replace extracellular volume
 • B. produce an osmotic diuresis
   C. block sodium reabsorbtion in the loop of Henle
   D. increase cardiac output

9. An oliguric patient is given 250 mg of furosemide intravenously and his urine output does not increase. This indicates he:
   A. most likely has ARF due to decreased renal perfusion
   B. requires fluid replacement

C. may have acute tubular necrosis (ATN)
   D. has developed uremic syndrome

10. Which of the following can contribute to hyperkalemia associated with ARF:
    A. kidney's decreased ability to excrete potassium
    B. metabolic acidosis due to inability to excrete acids
    C. catabolic state associated with severe illness
 • D. all of the above

11. Mrs. H. has ATN with oliguria. Her electrocardiogram shows sinus tachycardia with tall, tented T waves. Which of the following treatments would be most appropriate:
    A. administration of 200 mg furosemide
 • B. administration of Kayexalate and sorbitol
    C. administration of spironolactone
    D. initiation of a dopamine infusion

12. Mr. G. has ARF and is to be dialyzed in eight hours. Currently he is receiving intravenous glucose and insulin to correct:
    A. hyperglycemia associated with diabetes mellitus
    B. metabolic acidosis
 • C. hyperkalemia
    D. his serum calcium

13. Mrs. S. has been in the diuretic phase of ARF for several days. She has been experiencing personality changes and has just had a siezure. Which of the following actions would be the most appropriate in treating her problem:
    A. emergency peritoneal dialysis
 • B. infusion of a 3% sodium chloride solution
    C. administration of sodium bicarbonate
    D. infusion of a 5% dextrose in water (D5W) solution

124

14. Mrs. K. has been oliguric for 5 days and is complaining of nausea, anorexia, and vomiting. She has also developed a pericardial friction rub. These signs and symptoms can be attributed to:
    A. hyperkalemia
    B. an elevated serum creatinine
    C. hypermagnesemia
    • D. elevated blood urea nitrogen levels

15. Which of the following drugs should be avoided or have it's dosage reduced in the patient with renal failure:
    A. digitalis
    B. milk of magnesia
    C. cefazolin
    • D. all of the above

CHAPTER 26

Renal Transplantation

BEHAVIORAL OBJECTIVES

Based on the content in this chapter, the reader should be able to:

1. Define end-stage renal disease (ESRD).

2. Describe the altered body functions created by ESRD.

3. Compare and contrast the degrees to which dialysis and transplant manage various alterations created by ESRD.

4. List the criteria for selecting a kidney donor.

5. Recognize the signs and symptoms of postoperative transplantation complications including acute and chronic rejection, infection and altered urinary output.

6. Describe the immunosuppression drug therapy regimes.

7. Develop care plans for the pretransplant, postoperative and long-term phases of the transplantation process.

OVERVIEW

Chapter 26 begins by describing endstage renal disease and the resulting multisystem alterations. These are also summarized in an inclusive table. The major portion of the chapter explores renal transplantation. Indications and evaluation are the first steps in the process, followed by donor selection. Both living and cadaveric donation is explained along with issues involved in obtaining donors.

There is a thorough presentation of the assessment and management during the pre- and postoperative phases. Key points in postoperative care include monitoring the urinary function of the transplanted kidney, maintaining fluid and electrolyte balance and providing immunosuppressive therapy. The section on complications examines rejection and preventing life threatening infections and hypertension. A care plan is included.

KEY TERMS

histocompatibility	haplotype
human leukocyte antigens	

TEACHING/CLINICAL STRATEGIES

1. Arrange an observation experience on the kidney transplantation unit for selected students who can then share their experience with other students in clinical conference.

2. Arrange for student(s) to attend kidney transplantation nursing rounds and share

key points in clinical conference.

3. In conference have students compare the clinical findings, management, complications and rehabilitation for patients who have undergone either heart or kidney transplantation. Also compare the immunosuppressive regimes.

4. Arrange for a kidney transplant nurse specialist to present a conference on the care of patients undergoing kidney transplantation.

5. Arrange for a transplant coordinator to discuss the issues involved in obtaining donors. Have students dialogue with the coordinator on these issues and also discuss how they can approach a family about organ donation in the CCU when a patient is not expected to survive.

6. Have students read the research article cited in Chapter 26 as well as other articles on patient response to transplantation and discuss the implications for nurse interventions.

TEST QUESTIONS

1. A patient is considered to have end-stage renal disease (ESRD) when glomerular filtration rate decreases to:
   A. 0 ml/min
   • B. 10 ml/min
   C. 50 ml/min
   D. 100 ml/min

2. Renal osteodystrophy is caused by:
   A. lack of phosphorous
   B. elevated levels of serum magnesium
   C. decreased survival of red blood cells
   • D. decreased ability to activate vitamin D

3. Which of the following actions will help minimize renal osteodystrophy:
   A. administration of calcium carbonate
   B. dietary restriction of calcium and phosphorous
   C. administration of a synthetic form of activated vitamin D
   • D. all of the above

4. Which of the following occurs more often in the transplant patient than the dialysis patient with ESRD:
   A. renal osteodystrophy
   • B. gastric ulceration
   C. pulmonary edema
   D. impotence

5. In order to meet requirements for donor - recipient compatibility, which of the following is necessary:
   A. a positive crossmatch
   B. a two-haplotype match
   • C. red blood cell compatibility
   D. all of the above

6. An identical match of human leukocyte antigens (HLA) is most likely to occur in:
   • A. siblings
   B. parent and child
   C. husband and wife
   D. non-related donor and recipient

7. Which of the following patients could be a potential cadaveric kidney donor:
   • A. the trauma patient with a head injury
   B. the patient with metastasized lung cancer
   C. the trauma victim with sepsis
   D. all of the above

8. Mr. K. has just received a renal transplant this morning. His urinary catheter is draining bloody urine. This:
   A. indicates post-transplant acute tubular necrosis (ATN)
   B. is characteristic of organ rejection
   C. is due to leakage at the anastamosis site
   • D. is a normal finding

128

9. Which of the following is true regarding post-transplant ATN:
    A. it can be caused by prolonged preservation time
    B. it can be due to hypotensive periods experienced by the donor prior to death
    C. it is usually reversible
  • D. all of the above

10. Post-transplant diuresis is considered:
    A. a sign of ATN
  • B. to be due to a proximal tubular defect
    C. an indication of graft rejection
    D. a sign of normal graft functioning

11. Bone marrow suppression is a side effect of:
  • A. azathioprine
    B. methylprednisolone
    C. cyclosporine
    D. all of the above

12. Which of the following drugs is potentially nephrotoxic:
    A. methylprednisolone
    B. monoclonal antibody muromonab-CD3
  • C. cyclosporine
    D. antithymocyte globulin (ATG)

13. Mrs. R. had a cadaver transplant 2 weeks ago. She is complaining of fever, malaise, and tenderness over her graft site. Her serum creatinine and blood urea nitrogen (BUN) have been slowly increasing. Serum and urine beta-2 microglobulin are elevated. She is experiencing:
    A. hyperacute rejection
    B. accelerated rejection
  • C. acute rejection
    D. chronic rejection

14. You are caring for a post-transplant patient suffering from steroid induced hypertension. She may respond best to:
    A. propranolol
  • B. spironolactone
    C. minoxidi
    D. captopril

15. Mr. N. is a post-transplant patient. He has recently developed hypertension and a abdominal bruit heard medial to the kidney, but lateral to the midline. His treatment will most likely include:
    A. discontinuation of immunosuppressives
    B. an increase in his methylprednisolone dose
  • C. balloon angioplasty of the renal artery
    D. administration of spironolactone

CHAPTER 27

Anatomy and Physiology of the Nervous System

BEHAVIORAL OBJECTIVES

Based on the content in this chapter, the reader should be able to:

1. List the cellular units of the nervous system.

2. Briefly explain the physiology of a nerve impulse.

3. List two functions of cerebrospinal fluid (CSF).

4. Explain the functions of the thalamus.

5. Define the reticular activating system.

6. Briefly define the sensory system and the motor system.

7. List and explain three cord reflexes.

8. Explain the physiology of pain and the gate theory of pain regulation.

OVERVIEW

Chapter 27 presents an overview of the nervous system. Beginning with the cellular unit, the transmission of the nerve impulse is traced from the periphery to the central nervous system. Axons, dendrites, synapse, ganglia, nerve fiber covering and their regeneration are discussed along with neurotransmitters and threshold stimulus. Each component of the CNS structure and function are described. Cerebrospinal fluid, sensory and motor systems and cord reflexes are covered. Nerve pathways are explained along with both sympathetic and parasympathetic controls. The concepts involving cord reflexes, withdrawal, crossed extensive and peritoneal reflexes are discussed. Theories of pain are covered along with the description of endogenous opiates.

KEY TERMS

neuroglias	bulboreticular formation
Shwann cells	Gate theory
neurilemma	enkephalins
nodes of Ranvier	endorphins
fiber regeneration	referred pain
subarachnoid plexus	
basal ganglia	
Edinger-Westphal nucleus	

TEACHING/CLINICAL STRATEGIES

1. During class and conferences review the structure and function of the nervous system which relates to specific neurological injuries/illness.

2. When discussing bladder and bowel training apply content on spinal cord pathways and reflexes.

3. When students are practicing the neurological exam review the physiology of the structure being examined.

TEST QUESTIONS

1. Choose the most correct description of neurons.
    A. neurons have the ability to multiply and reproduce
  - B. neurons are the basic functional unit of the nervous system
    C. there are approximately 1 billion neurons in the CNS
    D. neurons connect to each other via myelin sheaths

2. In order for an action potential (or depolarization) to occur in a neuron:
  - A. there must be intact sodium-potassium pumps in the neuronal membrane
    B. there must be an influx of potassium into the cell
    C. there must be an electrical stimulus applied to the neuron
    D. the inside charge of the neuron must be positive in relation to the charge outside

3. The neurotransmitters involved in impulse conduction:
    A. include acetylcholine, epinephrine and dopamine
  - B. usually produce their effect by exciting the postsynaptic neuronal membrane
    C. are always inactivated by enzymes present in the synaptic cleft
    D. can stimulate both the pre and post ganglionic plates

4. Cerebrospinal fluid:
    A. is produced by the subarachnoid plexus
    B. is different from plasma in composition
    C. drains into the general circulation via the foramen magnum
  - D. acts to protect the CNS tissue and functions in the exchange of nutrients

5. You are preparing Mr. L. for a spinal tap. Because the spinal cord does not run the entire length of the spinal canal you know that the puncture is safer to perform at which level?
   A. T12 to L1 area
   B. below L5
   • C. below L2
   D. above L1

6. Verbal communication is an example of this level of brain function:
   A. mid brain
   B. medulla
   • C. cerebral cortex
   D. cerebellum

7. Your patient is recovering from a CVA. He is mainly having difficulty with equilibrium and coordination. He most likely has damage to:
   • A. the basal ganglia
   B. the cortex
   C. the thalamus
   D. the spinal cord

8. The pupillary light reflex center, the Edinger-Westphal nucleus, is located in the:
   A. cerebellum
   B. cortex
   • C. mid brain
   D. optic nerve

9. Consciousness, alertness, and attention probably occur in large part due to the:
   A. limbic system
   B. stimulant effect of endorphins
   C. bulboreticular formation
   • D. reticular activating system

10. Damage to the spinothalamic pathway of the spinal cord will result in:
    • A. problems in pain and temperature sensation

B. motor paralysis on the opposite side
C. weakness in the lower extremities
D. abnormal pupillary reflexes

11. 80% of all parasympathetic activity occurs by way of the:
    A. cerebrum
    • B. vagus nerve
    C. pelvic nerve
    D. spinal cord

12. Spinal cord reflexes occur without any control from higher brain centers. They include the:
    A. withdrawal from pain reflex
    B. stretch reflex (knee jerk)
    C. peritoneal reflex
    • D. all of the above

13. The gate theory about pain proposes that the amount of pain impulses reaching the brain are regulated in the:
    A. cerebellum
    B. spinothalamic fibers of the cord
    • C. substantia gelatinosa of the spinal cord
    D. none of the above

14. Referred pain, pain that is perceived as arising from a site that is not its true point of origin is:
    A. largely due to axonal connections between the 2 sites
    • B. probably the result of common embryologic tissue development of the 2 sites
    C. unpredictable and therefore of little concern
    D. due to crossing fibers in the spinal cord

CHAPTER **28**

Assessment: Nervous System

CHAPTER OUTLINE

Behavioral Objectives

Description

History

What to Ask about

Physical Examination

Level of Consciousness

Movement, Strength, and Coordination

Reflexes

Pupillary Changes

Vital Signs

Crainal Nerves

Occular Signs in the Unconscious Patient

Doll's Eyes and Caloric Reflex

Sensation

Other Observations

Evaluation of Dysfunction in Patient's
Living Patterns

Neurodiagnostic Tests and Normal Values

Neuroradiological Techniques

Computerized Axial Tomography

Magnetic Resonance Imaging (Mri)

Positron Emmision Tomography and
Single Photon Emmision Computerized
Tomography

Angiography and Digital Subtraction
Angiography

Myelography

Electrophysiological Studies

Electroencephalogram

Evoked Potentials

Transcranial Doppler Sonography

Lumbar Puncture and Csf Examination

Persistent Vegetative State

Brain Death

Study Questions

BEHAVIORAL OBJECTIVES

Based on the content in this chapter, the reader
should be able to:

1. Discuss the value of gathering
neurological data in an orderly and
objective manner.

2. Correlate such data over time.

3. Recognize those patterns of assessment
findings that imply a significant change in
pathology for the patient.

4. Relate the procedure of selected
neurodiagnostic tests to nursing
implication for patient care.

5. Evaluate the effect of neurological
dysfunction on the patient's living
patterns.

6. Define brain death.

OVERVIEW

Chapter 28 provides a clear, indepth

assessment of the nervous system. The assessment purpose is to provide systematic, objective information that can be correlated over time and will help determine the effect of the dysfunction on self care. The physical examination section explores levels of consciousness, movement, strength and coordination, pupil response, ocular signs, sensation and activities of daily living. Testing each cranial nerve is described. Pertinent assessment tools illustrate each part of the neuro exam. Examples of tools include the Glascow Coma Scale and the stimulus reaction scale.

Ten diagnostic tests are explained along with the nursing responsibilities for patient and family preparation and patient monitoring. A table summarizes key points about neurodiagnostic testing, such as purpose, data provided, and nursing implications. Persistent vegetative state with its lack of apparent recognition is described along with brain death.

KEY TERMS

obtunded	agnosia
stuporous	stereognosis
adiadokokinesia	graphesthesia
decorticate	point localization
decerebrate	extinction
deep tendon reflexes (DVT)	phenomenon
Romberg Test	two-point discrimination
Rapidly Alternating Movement (RAM)	texture discrimination
quadrant deficit	Battle's sign
oculocephalic reflex	Raccoon's eye
oculovestibular reflex	rhinorrhea
	otorrhea

meningeal irritation

TEACHING/CLINICAL STRATEGIES

1. Have students practice the neuro examination on each other in the laboratory and then examine their patients who require nervous system assessment.

2. Have students participate in preparing a patient and family for neurodiagnostic testing, accompany the patient and participate in posttest monitoring.

3. Arrange for students to attend nursing rounds for patients with neuro system problems.

4. Arrange clinical experience for students in which they care for patients who require neuro system assessment.

5. Arrange for a clinical specialist to demonstrate the neuro assessment and discuss how the findings help determine nursing and medical management.

TEST QUESTIONS

1. One of the most critical parameters in the neurologic assessment is:
   A. visual field evaluation
   B. memory
   C. the Romberg test
   • D. level of consciousness

2. Mr. J. is a 60 year old patient who had a cerebral aneurysm repaired. Immediately post-op he opens his eyes to noxious stimuli, has garbled speech, and withdraws from painful stimuli. His Glascow Coma Score would be:
   • A. 8
   B. 11
   C. 5
   D. 13

3. When assessing movement, strength and coordination, the nurse notes that the patient has twitching of muscles while at rest. This type of involuntary movement is called:
   A. tremors
   B. clonus
   • C. fasiculations
   D. none of the above

4. Ms. K. has been in a motor vehicle crash and is in the critical care unit with a severe brain injury. She is comatose but when painful stimuli is applied she extends, adducts and hyperpronates her upper extremities and has plantar flexion of the feet. This abnormal response is termed:
   A. decorticate rigidity
   • B. decerebrate rigidity
   C. clonic-tonic activity
   D. athetosis

5. In assessing for pupillary changes, the nurse includes evaluation of:
   • A. size, shape, and reaction to light and accommodation
   B. size, shape, and corneal reflex
   C. size, shape and visual acuity
   D. none of the above

6. The classic signs of increased intracranial pressure include:
   A. dilated pupils, hypotension, tachycardia
   • B. elevated systolic pressure, widened pulse pressure, bradycardia, respiratory irregularities
   C. respiratory irregularities, elevated systolic pressure, tachycardia
   D. none of the above

7. The nurse is observing the oculovestibular reflex (caloric test). A normal response involves:
   A. the eyes do not move in response to the stimulus
   B. the pupils dilate in response to the stimulus
   • C. the eyes exhibit nystagmus and slowly move toward the side of the stimulus
   D. the eyes exhibit nystagmus and then rotate upward

8. The oculocephalic and oculovestibular reflexes are tested in unconscious patients to determine:
   A. brain death
   • B. brainstem functioning
   C. level of coma
   D. cranial nerve function

9. Kernig's sign and Brudzinski's sign may indicate:
   A. herniation
   B. brain stem dysfunction
   C. brain death
   • D. meningeal irritation

10. Mr. L. is having a myelogram study to evaluate his back pain. Appropriate nursing care would include all except:
    A. keep head of bed elevated at least 30-45 degrees
    • B. restrict fluids
    C. avoid phenothiazine medications
    D. assure liberal fluid intake

11. Mrs. G. is a 32 year old woman who is in a persistent vegetative state after a car accident. As the nurse, you know that:
    A. Mrs. G. is brain dead
    • B. Mrs. G. may appear conscious, have voluntary movement, and sleep-wake patterns
    C. her condition will improve with time
    D. she still has higher cortical brain functioning

12. The role of the nurse in caring for a potentially brain dead patient includes:
    A. question the possibility of brain death
    B. assist in data gathering to determine brain death
    C. support the patient's family
    • D. all of the above

13. Mr. C. had a cerebral angiography, performed to evaluate his aneurysm. Appropriate post-procedure nursing interventions include all the following except:
    A. assess puncture site for swelling, bleeding, redness
    B. assure adequate fluid intake
    C. assess limb distal to puncture site for pulses, color, and temperature
    • D. ambulate frequently

CHAPTER **29**

```
┌─────────────────────────────────┐
│                                 │
│  *Management Modalities:*       │
│  *Nervous System*               │
│                                 │
└─────────────────────────────────┘
```

Management Modalities: Nervous System

BEHAVIORAL OBJECTIVES

Based on the content in this section, the reader should be able to:

1. Identify four indications for intracranial pressure (ICP) monitoring.

2. List four techniques for obtaining ICP measurements.

3. Define cerebral perfusion pressure (CPP).

4. Describe three interventions used to promote adequate cerebral blood flow (CBF) in the presence of increased intracranial pressure (IICP).

5. List three possible nursing diagnoses for the patient with IICP and describe the nursing interventions for each diagnosis.

Section B: Hypothermia

SECTION OUTLINE

BEHAVIORAL OBJECTIVES

Based on the content in this section, the reader should be able to:

1. Explain the rationale for using induced hypothermia in a clinical situation.

2. List and explain two methods for inducing hypothermia in the clinical setting.

3. Identify 3 causes of unintentional (accidental) hypothermia.

4. Describe three nursing diagnoses and their appropriate nursing interventions for the hypothermic patient.

OVERVIEW

Intracranial pressure monitoring and hypothermia are the two management modalities presented in this chapter.

Intracranial pressure monitoring explores intracranial dynamics that include the Nonro-Kelle hypothesis, autoregulation and the intracranial volume-pressure curve. Intracranial pressure (ICP) monitoring equipment and techniques are illustrated. The pros and cons for each technique are presented along with the indications for monitoring, pressure ranges, waveforms and their significance.

The use of ventilation, head elevation, hypothermia, blood pressure reduction and CSF drainage and their role in managing IICP are described. The use of pharmacologics such as steroids, osmotic agents, calcium antagonists and barbiturates (to induce coma) are also covered. The risks for infection, coagulopathy and sepsis are discussed. A care plan is included.

The next section describes the principles, purposes, techniques and nursing responsibilities for hypothermia. The body's response to hypothermia is explored along with physiological events that occur at certain temperatures. For example, coagulopathy, hypoglycemia, shivering and vital sign responses are explained. Warming and cooling systems are explained along with the procedure for cooling and rewarming. Monitoring temperature and vital body functions are described as well as nursing responsibilities for overseeing total patient care, preserving skin integrity and range of motion, and preventing pneumonia. A care plan is included.

KEY TERMS

intracranial pressure (ICP)

cerebral perfusion pressure (CCP)

volume-pressure curve

vasomotor paralysis

ventriculostomy

brain stem auditory

evoked response (BAER)

conduction

convection

core temperature

thermoregulation

thermoperception

TEACHING/CLINICAL STRATEGIES

1. Arrange for students to observe or participate in the care of patients having ICP monitoring or hypothermia.

2. Have clinical specialist demonstrate ICP monitoring and hypothermia equipment either in the CCU or in a simulated set up or by a video or slides.

3. In case conference have clinical specialist discuss patients who require either ICP monitoring or hypothermia illustrating key observations/findings and their implications.

TEST QUESTIONS

1. Intracranial pressure is:
   A. normal at 25-30 mmHg
   - B. determined by the amount of brain tissue, CSF, and blood
   C. equal to cerebral perfusion pressure (CPP)
   D. only measured during cranial surgery

2. The most potent cerebrovasodilator is:
   A. barbiturates
   B. morphine
   C. oxygen
   - D. carbon dioxide

3. While caring for a patient with increased intracranial pressure it is important that the nurse:
   A. keep the head of the bed flat
   B. maintain the hips in a flexed position
   - C. avoid neck and hip flexion
   D. keep the head of the bed elevated to 45 degrees

4. Cerebral perfusion pressure (CPP) is:
   A. equal to ICP-MAP
   B. normal at approximately 30 mmHg
   - C. affected by both blood pressure and ICP
   D. none of the above

5. A patient with an intraventricular catheter for ICP measurement should have the transducer placed:
   - A. near the tragus of the ear or at the edge of the eyebrow
   B. at the jawline
   C. under the scalp
   D. at the level of the right atrium

6. ICP waveforms:
   A. are not usually influenced by blood pressure or respiratory efforts
   - B. resemble arterial pressure or central venous pressure waveforms
   C. are seldom monitored due to their lack of clinical significance
   D. resemble R ventricular pressure waveforms

7. The nurse is caring for a patient with an ICP monitoring device in place and the waveform becomes flat. The nurse should:
   A. assume that the ICP has fallen and notify the physician
   B. flush with 10 cc normal saline
   - C. check for air in the tubing/transducer, check for disconnections in the system
   D. all of the above

8. When hyperventilating the patient to help control ICP, the usual ventilatory parameter used is:
   A. respiratory rate
   B. pH
   C. tidal volume
   - D. $PaCO_2$ level

9. Mr. J. is being hyperventilated to control his elevated ICP. His last ABGs show pH 7.50, PaO_2 90 mmHg, $PaCO_2$ 15 mmHg. The nurse should realize that:
   A. these values are within the therapeutic range
   - B. this $PaCO_2$ is lower than the therapeutic level and may be detrimental to the patient
   C. this $PaCO_2$ is higher than the therapeutic level and may not be affecting the ICP
   D. this pH reflects acidemia

10. Mrs. L. is in a barbiturate coma to control her ICP. Important nursing care activities include:
    A. frequent turning with passive ROM
    B. rigorous pulmonary care (suctioning, postural drainage)
    C. monitoring pentobarbital levels
    - D. all of the above

11. Hypothermia:
    A. is defined as a core temperature of less than 33°C
    B. may be beneficial with neurologic patients because it raises cerebral blood flow
    - C. may be beneficial with neurologic patients because it lowers the brain's metabolic rate
    D. is always an untoward effect of barbiturate coma

12. Mr. B. is an obese patient who has just had an evacuation of a subarachnoid hematoma. The post-op orders include "Use cooling blanket to keep temp. at 32°C." The nurse should:
    - A. turn the cooling blanket off before the patient's temp reaches 32°C

B. allow the patient's temp to get slightly lower than 32°C before removing the cooling blanket

C. use two cooling blankets

D. question this order as 32°C is much too low to maintain a temperature

13. Complications associated with hypothermia include all but:
   A. fat necrosis
   B. rewarming shock
   C. cardiac dysrhythmias
   • D. dehydration secondary to increased urine output

CHAPTER 30

Head Injury

CHAPTER OUTLINE

BEHAVIORAL OBJECTIVES

Based on the content in this chapter, the reader should be able to:

1. Identify possible mechanisms of head injury associated with trauma.

2. Describe various types of head injuries and their associated symptomatology.

3. Explain the pathophysiology of potential

4. Discuss the rationale for medical and nursing management in the therapy of the head-injured patient.

OVERVIEW

Chapter 30 describes the types, consequences, assessment and management of brain injuries. In order to understand the effects of brain injuries, the location, severity and mechanism are explained along with the secondary effects of hypoxia, hypercarbia, and hypotension. Skull fractures, concussions, contusion, hematomas and their accompanying findings; the likely timing of deterioration, and mortality rates are described. Pathophysiological principles explain the major impairments which include breathing, mobility, hydration, swallowing, cognition and communication. Respiratory and positioning patterns resulting from intracranial dysfunctions are discussed so the practitioner can begin to pick up clues early.

Management content presents nursing interventions and their rationale. Evaluating respiratory status, coughing and swallowing is explained in relation to determining when oral feeding can begin. Interventions which address abnormal posturing, hydration, elimination, feeding and communication problems are covered. A sensory stimulation plan is described in order to help the patient attend to selective environmental stimuli. Complications such as pulmonary edema, seizures, and CSF leak are explained. A case study and care plan are included.

KEY TERMS

shearing injury	diffuse injury
focal injury	concussion
contusion	capnography
Cheyne-Stokes breathing	opisthotonic posturing
central neurogenic hyperventilation	dysarthria
	apraxia
cluster breathing	
dysphagia	

CLINICAL/TEACHING STRATEGIES

1. Arrange for students to observe/participate in the care of patients' with brain injury.

2. Invite a representative from the area Traumatic Brain Injury Association to discuss statistics and preventive measures surrounding TBI.

3. In a lecture on head injury discuss the types of injuries, acute phase findings and their significance, and nursing responsibilities.

4. Lecture on some special nursing issues accompanying head injury. For example, discuss the nutritional requirements in the critical phase of injury evaluating swallowing and readiness for feeding. Invite speech therapist to participate. Discuss bladder and bowel elimination, cognition, and communication problems. Integrate concepts from Chapter 35 on nutritional assessment and Chapter 4 on sensory input.

5. Arrange demonstration of pressure relief beds.

6. Arrange for student(s) to attend grand rounds or interdisciplinary case conferences which discuss patients with head injury.

7. In conference, have students discuss their interactions with families. Integrate

concepts and learning activities from Chapter 3 Caring for the Patient's Family.

TEST QUESTIONS

1. The mechanism of head injury occurring in a fall is usually:
   A. an acceleration injury
   ● B. a deceleration injury
   C. coup-contrecoup injury
   D. none of the above

2. Basilar skull fractures:
   A. are the least significant type of skull fracture
   ● B. may cause CSF leaks from the nose or ears
   C. have no characteristic findings/signs
   D. are always surgically repaired

3. Mr. L. was hit in the head with a baseball bat. He had a brief loss of consciousness and presents to the emergency department alert and oriented x 3. Soon after, Mr. L. becomes unconscious. His injury is most likely:
   A. a subdural hematoma
   B. a coup-contrecoup injury
   C. an intracerebral bleed
   ● D. an epidural hematoma

4. Patients with a sub acute subdural hematoma will usually present with symptoms:
   ● A. 2 days to 2 weeks after injury
   B. 1 month after injury
   C. 24-48 hours after injury
   D. 3-4 months after injury

5. Mrs. B. has an intercerebral hematoma that is being managed medically. The nurse notes that Mrs. B. is exhibiting ataxic breathing. The nurse should:
   A. realize that all patients with head injury exhibit changes in respiratory patterns and not be alarmed
   ● B. notify the physician and make sure the equipment for intubation and ventilation are accessible

   C. insert a nasopharyngeal airway to suction the patient
   D. realize that this is indication of improved neurologic function

6. Mr. Z. has a severe brain injury and is exhibiting the following signs and symptoms: coma, decreased urine output, urine specific gravity of greater than 1.025, and decreased hematocrit. The nurse will:
   A. anticipate that Mr. Z is in Diabetes Insipidus (DI) and will expect to increase his fluid intake
   B. continue to monitor the patient, expecting no change in plans
   ● C. know that Mr. Z is most likely having SIADH, and will expect to restrict fluids and give diuretics
   D. irrigate the foley catheter and increase the IV rate

7. The nurse is caring for a head injured patient who is being evaluated for swallowing ability. The nurse knows that:
   A. patients may have trouble detecting the presence of food in their mouth
   B. thin fluids are more difficult to swallow than thick fluids
   C. swallowing is a 3 stage process involving multiple brain areas and cranial nerve reflexes
   ● D. all of the above

8. When suctioning a head injured patient it is important to:
   ● A. hyperoxygenate before, during and after to prevent secondary brain injury secondary to hypoxia and increased ICP
   B. suction the nasopharynx of all patients
   C. increase the tidal volume prior to suctioning
   D. turn the head from side to side to facilitate L bronchus suctioning

9. One of the primary nursing responsibilities in caring for the brain injured comatose patient is:
   A. planning for early rehabilitation
   B. family education regarding prognosis and long term care
   • C. prevent skin problems by preventing pressure
   D. early initiation of bowel and bladder program

10. Mrs. K. is 3 days post-op after having an epidural hematoma evacuated. While the nurse is in the room Mrs. K. has a generalized seizure. The nurse should do all the following except:
   A. turn Mrs. K. to her side
   B. help maintain a patent airway
   • C. pry open Mrs. K.'s jaws to place a padded tongue blade between her teeth
   D. restrain Mrs. K.'s movements only enough to prevent her from hurting herself

CHAPTER **31**

Common Neurological Disorders

BEHAVIORAL OBJECTIVES

Based on the content in this chapter, the reader should be able to:

1. Name three common clinical manifestations of a right hemispheric stroke.

2. Name three common clinical manifestations of a left hemispheric stroke.

3. Discuss two treatment modalities available for the patient with an arteriovenous formation; a cerebral aneurysm.

4. Describe three appropriate nursing interventions for a patient with a cerebral aneurysm prior to surgery.

5. Describe four observations to be made

during a seizure.

6. Discuss three important facts a patient taking phenytoin should be taught.

7. Differentiate between partial and generalized seizures.

8. Explain the pathophysiology of Guillan-Barre syndrome.

9. Formulate a teaching plan for a patient with myasthenia gravis.

OVERVIEW

Chapter 31 covers six neurological disorders and integrates concepts from earlier chapters. The first disorder, cerebrovascular disease, presents information important for nurses caring for patients at any level of acuity. The types of strokes, pathology and resulting symptoms, progress predictors and resulting neurological deficits are described. Management explains drugs and tests to control and monitor vasospasm, anticoagulation, hypertension and increased intracranial pressure. Tests which monitor cerebral circulation and oxygenation are described. Ways to prevent complications from immobility and manage emotions, behavior and communication problems are addressed.

The section on arteriovenous malformations describes the congenital defects, course and management of hemorrhage. The section on cerebral aneurysms gives an overview of the course and survival rates, clinical manifestations and severity grading. The use of transcranial doppler ultrasonography for diagnosis and vasospasm monitoring is explained. Management covers drug treatment, and surgical excision and postoperative course. Nursing management presents patient/family education and neurological monitoring. Complications address treating vasospasm by hypervolemia and hemodilution; and nursing responsibilities in monitoring hemodynamic pressures, pulmonary edema and increased intracranial pressure. A case study and care plan are included.

The section on seizure disorders describes the pathophysiology of paroxysmal depolarization shifts, generalized and focal seizures and their symptoms. Assessing seizures addresses eleven areas to observe and record. The need for thoughtful diagnosis by CT, MRI and metabolic workup is covered as well as treatment by atiepileptic drugs, microsurgery and implantable neurocybernetic prosthesis. Areas for patient and family teaching are detailed. Coping mechanisms, psychosocial problems and possible personality disorders which may occur from long term seizure problems are included.

The section on Guillain Barre Syndrome presents the pathophysiology and clinical course. Management explains the use of plasma phoresis and potential complications, and focuses on the issues of sleep deprivation secondary to increased nocturnal muscle pain, the risk of respiratory failure and the need for emotional support. A case study and care plan are included.

The last section addresses the incidence, pathophysiology, diagnostic tests and clinical findings of myasthenia gravis. Management explores medication therapy with anticholinesterates, steroids and immunosuppressive drugs along with athymectomy or plasma phoresis. Complications describe the symptoms and treatment for both myasthenic and cholinergic crises.

KEY TERMS

stroke in evolution

completed stroke

arteriovenous malformation (AVM)

reversible ischemic neurological deficit (RIND)

saturation of jugular oxygen (SjO2)

arteriovenous difference of oxygen (AVDO2)

transcranial doppler ultrasonography (TCD)

triple H therapy

paroxysmal depolarization shifts (PDS)

generalized seizure

focal or partial seizure

pseudoseizure

antiepileptic drugs (AED)

neurocybernetic prosthesis (NCP)

plasma phoresis

transcutaneous electrical stimulus (TEN's)

electromyography

TEACHING/CLINICAL STRATEGIES

1. Arrange for students to participate/observe care of patients with neurological crises.

2. Conduct a class in which the nursing management of patients with neurological disorders is compared and contrasted.

3. Invite a clinical specialist to present case examples which demonstrate key pathophysiology, clinical findings, and nursing management concepts.

4. In clinical conference have students discuss the patients they have cared for and apply principles of neurological assessment including cranial nerve and LOC evaluation, and ICP monitoring.

5. Arrange for students to attend grand rounds or an interdisciplinary case conference for patients with acute neurological disorders.

6. In conference have students share their interactions with patients and families and discuss both patient and family response to illness. Refer to concepts in Chapters 2 & 3.

TEST QUESTIONS

1. Cerebrovascular disease (CVD), due to thrombosis, embolism, or hemorrhage:
   A. results in the same ischemic insult to the brain
   B. is the 3rd leading cause of morbidity and mortality in adults in the U.S.
   C. is the most frequent neurologic disorder in adults
   • D. all of the above

2. Cerebral vascular accidents (CVAs) are:
   • A. most often due to thrombi or emboli
   B. never preventable
   C. usually associated with decreased level of consciousness
   D. all of the above

3. Mr. C. is in the ICU after a CVA. He has a jugular catheter in place to monitor venous oxygenation saturation in blood returning from the cerebral hemispheres. The nurse needs to know that:
   A. this catheter should be flushed periodically
   B. normal jugular oxygen saturation is 60-80%
   C. this is still an investigational monitoring technique
   • D. all of the above

4. The most common complications associated with subarachnoid hemorrhage are:
   A. hypoxia, seizures, pupil changes
   • B. vasospasm, hydrocephalus, dysrhythmias
   C. vasospasm, seizures, behavior changes
   D. none of the above

5. J. K. is a 20 year old male in the ICU with the diagnosis of AVM. The nurse should be aware that:
   - A. seizure activity may occur
   - B. hemorrhage of the AVM is rare
   - C. having this diagnosis at a young age carries a poor prognosis
   - D. the management will most frequently be medical in nature

6. When a cerebral aneurysm ruptures, patients may experience all of the following except:
   - A. severe headache
   - B. cardiac dysrhythmias and hypertension
   - C. hypovolemic shock
   - D. localized neurologic deficits

7. Pharmacologic management of ruptured cerebral aneurysm may include:
   - A. Amicar
   - B. stool softeners
   - C. calcium antagonists
   - D. all of the above

8. Mr. P. is in the ICU after a ruptured cerebral aneurysm. During the nurse's assessment it is noted that Mr. P. has new onset of hemiparesis, is slightly lethargic and difficult to arouse, and when awake complains of diploplia. These symptoms suggest:
   - A. a rebleed of the aneurysm
   - B. increased ICP
   - C. vasospasm
   - D. carbon dioxide retention

9. The nurse caring for an unconscious patient should be aware that:
   - A. talking about that person at the bedside will cause a rise in ICP
   - B. all procedures should be explained regardless of level of consciousness
   - C. the patient may be able to hear and understand conversation
   - D. all of the above

10. Mrs. L. has just returned to the ICU after having a cerebral aneurysm clipped. The most important parameter that the nurse should assess is:
    - A. pupillary response to light
    - B. gag reflex
    - C. extremity movement and sensation
    - D. level of consciousness

11. The major treatment modalities for vasospasm include:
    - A. hypervolemia, induced hypertension, hemodilution
    - B. hypotension, hypovolemia, hemoconcentration
    - C. pain management, Amicar, calcium channel blockers
    - D. none of the above

12. Pseudo seizures can usually be differentiated from generalized tonicclonic seizures in that pseudo seizures usually do not include:
    - A. tonic-clonic movements
    - B. incontinence and cyanosis
    - C. incontinence and tongue-biting
    - D. injury to the patient

13. When administering phenytoin for control of seizures the nurse must be aware that:
    - A. phenytoin will precipitate in dextrose solutions
    - B. it should be given at a rate of 40-50 mg/min.
    - C. cardiac dysrhythmias or hypotension may occur
    - D. all of the above

14. Guillain-Barre Syndrome is frequently associated with:
    - A. descending paralysis/weakness
    - B. history of a recent viral infection
    - C. seizures
    - D. all of the above

15. Myasthenia Gravis is a neuromuscular disorder thought to be due to:

- A. a reduction in the number of functioning acetylcholine receptors at the neuromuscular junction
  B. loss of myelin along the nerves
  C. a viral infection
  D. the presence of an antibody at the nerve synapse which blocks the neurotransmitter dopamine

Chapter 32

Spinal Cord Injury

BEHAVIORAL OBJECTIVES

Based on the content in this chapter, the reader should be able to:

1. Differentiate between a complete and an incomplete spinal cord injury (SCI).

2. Explain the pathophysiology involved with a Brown-Sequard syndrome, a central cord syndrome and an anterior cord syndrome.

3. Describe three clinical features of spinal shock.

4. Describe two immediate nursing actions to take after autonomic dysreflexia is recognized.

5. Develop a holistic care plan for a patient with an acute spinal cord injury.

OVERVIEW

Chapter 32 covers spinal cord injury through the primary, secondary and tertiary stages of recovery. After a description of the statistics, causes and consequences of injuries, pathophysiological principles explore various levels of spinal cord injuries and the resulting motor and sensory impairments. These concepts are expanded in the assessment section which describes multiple body system findings. An initial assessment determines the extent of spinal cord and accompanying injuries. Diagnostic studies and the significance of the digital rectal exam are discussed. The signs, symptoms and consequences for the respiratory system, metabolic depression and spinal cord shock are examined along with the importance of maintaining a positive nitrogen balance.

The management section includes medical, collaborative and nursing management. Medical management for each body system is discussed beginning with hemodynamic stability, cord decompression and immobilization, and respiratory maintenance. Collaborative management focuses on preventing DVT, maintaining body temperature and providing urinary continence, along with a straightforward discussion on maintaining sexual activity. Nursing management provides a thorough discussion of bowel and bladder training, skin care and preventing respiratory complications. Potential complications throughout recovery are discussed and include stress ulcers, autonomic reflexia and contractures in the acute phase; and hypercalcemia, spinal cord ischemia and substance abuse in the later phases. A case study and a care plan are included.

KEY TERMS

dermatomes	syndrome
quadriplegia	spinal shock
central cord syndrome	quad coughing techniques
Brown-Sequard syndrome	digital stimulation
ipsilaterally	autonomic dysreflexia
anterior cord	gastro-colic reflex

TEACHING/CLINICAL STRATEGIES

1. Arrange for students to observe/participate in the care of patients with spinal cord injury.

2. Invite a clinical specialist to discuss patient situations and the issues surrounding their care throughout the early phase of recovery.

3. Arrange for students to attend interdisciplinary case conferences about

patients recovering from spinal cord injury.

4. In conference discuss students interactions with patients about their response to the injury. Integrate concepts from Chapter 2 Psychosocial Concepts and the Patient's Experience with Critical Illness.

5. In conference have students discuss their interactions with families. Integrate concepts and learning activities from Chapter 3 Caring for the Patient's Family.

TEST QUESTIONS

1. One of the most important assessment parameters in the initial management of a patient with spinal cord injury (SCI) is:
   A. bowel function and rectal tone
   B. sensation and movement of extremities
   - C. lung sounds and tidal volume measurements
   D. deep tendon reflexes

2. J.L. is a 19 year old patient with a C5-6 SCI. On day 2 in the ICU the nurse notes that the patient has decreased urine output. The nurse knows that:
   A. this indicates that the patient is hypovolemic
   - B. this may be a part of the metabolic response to injury
   C. this is most likely the result of the lack of innervation to the bladder
   D. none of the above

3. A patient with spinal shock will manifest which of the following signs/symptoms?
   A. hypertension, headache, flushing
   - B. hypotension, bradycardia, lack of deep tendon reflexes
   C. hypotension, tachycardia, loss of sensation
   D. diaphoresis, flushing, tachycardia

4. C.G. is a 17 year old patient with a C3-4 fracture and cord injury. The nurse will anticipate that C.G.:
   - A. will be ventilator dependent
   B. will be able to be independent of the ventilator
   C. will need a manual wheelchair
   D. none of the above

5. Current studies are being undertaken to determine the effectiveness of a new drug therapy for SCI. This drug is:
   A. Heparin
   B. Ibuprofen
   - C. Solumedrol
   D. Interferon

6. J.L., a patient with a T3-4 SCI, is in the ICU. Shortly after his bath the nurse notes he is hypertensive, flushed, and he complains of a severe headache. The nurse should:
   A. do nothing, this response will pass
   B. lower the head of the bed and notify the physician
   - C. raise the head of the bed, check the bladder drainage system for kinks, check for bowel impaction
   D. increase the IV fluid rate and clamp the urinary catheter

7. During an intermittent catheterization program, the patient should be taught to:
   - A. empty the bladder using the Crede or Valsalva maneuver
   B. catheterize every 2 hours
   C. increase fluid intake between catheterizations
   D. stop catheterization when residuals are less than 350 cc

8. A.K. has a T6 SCI. She is difficult to work with because she has unrealistic expectations that she will one day walk. She is denying that her injury is permanent. The best approach for the nurse to take is:
   A. encourage her hopes, she may be right

B. focus on long term life changes she will be facing

C. listen and firmly redirect her expectations

- D. focus on her present problems

9. Intramuscular injections in SCI patients should be:

    A. given in the deltoid or abdominal area

    B. limited to 1 cc of volume

    C. used with caution as the medication may not be absorbed well

- D. all of the above

10. The preferred intravenous site in the acute management of SCI patients is:

    A. a peripheral lower extremity vein

- B. the subclavian vein

    C. the femerol vein

    D. none of the above

11. J.D. is a 34 year old patient with an SCI. After two months in the hospital J.D. expresses concern to the nurse that she hasn't had a menstrual period since her accident. The nurse explains that:

- A. it may take approximately 6 months for her periods to return

    B. she will probably not have a normal menstrual cycle

    C. she will most likely not have periods and will not need birth control

    D. she should have started her periods by now and she'll report this to the physician

12. When caring for a patient in a halo brace it is important to:

    A. keep the wrench taped to vest for quick removal for CPR

    B. check skull pin tightness every day

    C. discourage use of pillow under ring

- D. all of the above

CHAPTER **33**

Anatomy and Physiology of the Gastrointestinal System

CHAPTER OUTLINE

BEHAVIORAL OBJECTIVES

Based on the content in this chapter, the reader should be able to:

1. List three major functions of the gastrointestinal system.

2. Outline the result of each digestive organ's secretion and processing of substrates.

3. Describe the breakdown of carbohydrates, proteins, fats and vitamins.

4. Outline the events that occur during emesis.

5. Identify three steps in the process of defecation.

6. List five important functions of the liver.

OVERVIEW

This chapter presents content which serves as a foundation for understanding this unit as well as the endocrine unit. Each part of the digestive system is examined from a structural and physiological perspective. Motility, circulation, innervation, secretions and absorption are discussed. Some key points to consider involve events surrounding swallowing, digestion, emesis, defecation and the effects of emotion on this system. The multiple functions of the liver are also explored. Discussion of the pancreas is begun here and expanded in the endocrine section. Tables summarize digestion, secretions and absorption, and hepatic functions.

KEY TERMS

lower esophageal sphincter

submucosa

Peyer's patches

cholinergic blockers

intrinsic factor

cephalic phase

gastric phase

intestinal phase

acinar cells

hepatocytes

commensal bacteria

TEACHING/CLINICAL STRATEGIES

1. During clinical conference discuss critically ill patients who have problems with constipation, diarrhea or bowel incontinence. Discuss the factors related to these nursing diagnoses, the physiological processes which have been interrupted and nursing interventions.

2. In clinical conferences, have students identify the side effects of medications on the GI tract, including the liver, and describe the way in which the medications interfere with normal physiology.

3. In class or conference, integrate the physiological concepts of the pancreas and liver when discussing pancreatitis and hepatic disorders.

TEST QUESTIONS

1. Sympathetic stimulation of the gastrointestinal tract results in:
   A. decreased tonicity of sphincters
   B. increased pancreatic secretions
   • C. decreased motility
   D. an increase in saliva production

2. Amylase is secreted by the:
   A. pancreas
   B. parotid gland
   C. submaxillary salivary gland
   • D. all of the above

3. Esophogeal cells secrete:
   • A. mucus
   B. saliva
   C. amylase
   D. digestive enzymes

4. Hydrochloric acid (HCl):
   A. is secreted by chief cells in the stomach
   B. secretion is stimulated by intrinsic factor
   • C. is necessary to activate pepsinogen
   D. all of the above

5. Following a vagotomy:
   A. gastrin secretion would be reduced
   • B. HCL would not be secreted in response to the smell of food
   C. gastric emptying is enhanced
   D. parietal cell secretions would be reduced during the gastric phase of secretion regulation

6. HCl secretion can be stimulated by:
   A. histamine antagonists
   B. prostaglandins
 • C. alcohol
   D. all of the above

7. The pancreas secretes:
   A. potassium
   B. bicarbonate
   C. digestive enzymes
 • D. all of the above

8. Proteins entering the duodenum are digested by:
   A. lipase
 • B. trypsin
   C. amylase
   D. gastrin

9. Which of the following substances is necessary for fat absorption:
   A. amylase
   B. chymotrypsin
   C. HCl
 • D. bile

10. Which of the following substances are reabsorbed in the colon:
    A. bile salts and fat
    B. nutrients
 • C. water and potassium
    D. vitamins and minerals

11. The liver helps maintain colloid osmotic pressure by the:
    A. conversion of ammonia to urea

 • B. synthesis of albumin
   C. elimination of bilirubin
   D. release of glucose into plasma

12. Failure of the liver to degrade steroid hormones can result in:
    A. a build up of ammonia in the blood
 • B. excess blood levels of aldosterone
    C. insufficient blood levels of estrogen
    D. the development of ascites

13. The liver can raise plasma glucose levels when stimulated by:
 • A. growth hormone
    B. insulin
    C. aldosterone
    D. secretin

14. An obstruction of the duct of Wirsung can lead to:
    A. bile accumulation in the Ampulla of Vater
    B. back up of bile into the gallbladder
 • C. inability of pancreatic secretions to empty into the duodenum
    D. back up of pancreatic secretions and bile into the pancreas

15. Gallbladder contraction can be stimulated by:
    A. duodenal peristalsis
    B. enterokinase
    C. built up pressure behind the duct of Wirsung
 • D. the parasympathetic nervous system

CHAPTER **34**

Assessment: Gastrointestinal System

CHAPTER OUTLINE

Behavioral Objectives

Description

History

Physical Examination

  Oral Cavity

  Abdominal Examination

    Observation

    Auscultation

    Percussion

    Palpation

  Rectal Examination

  Documentation

  Ongoing Assessment

Diagnostic Tests

  X-rays

  Gastroendoscopy

  Colonoscopy

  Barium Contrast Studies

  Ultrasonography

  Computed Axial Tomography

  Arteriography

  Paracentesis

Management

  Preprocedure Care

  Postprocedure Care

Study Questions

BEHAVIORAL OBJECTIVES

Based on the content in this chapter, the reader should be able to:

1. Identify the basic components of a nursing history in assessing the gastrointestinal system.

2. Name the five features assessed in a review of the gastrointestinal system.

3. Describe a basic examination of the oral cavity using inspection and palpation.

4. Describe a physical examination of the abdomen and specific modifications used during inspection, auscultation, percussion and palpation.

5. Describe two nursing interventions for patients undergoing endoscopic and radiographic studies of the gastrointestinal tract.

OVERVIEW

This chapter describes the principles involved in history taking and physical examination of the GI system. A systems review highlights the most common complaints, including pain and accompanying psychological factors.

The examination covers general appearance, head, skin and abdomen. The abdominal exam describes inspection, auscultation, percussion and palpation. A documentation sample is included. Seven diagnostic tests are explained along with pre and postprocedure care.

KEY TERMS

gastrointestinal endoscopy

endoscopic retrograde cholangiopan-creatography

colonoscopy

ultrasonography

computed axial tomography

TEACHING/CLINICAL STRATEGIES

1. Have students prepare and accompany their patients who are having gastrointestinal diagnostic tests.

2. Have students practice abdominal examination on each other in the laboratory and then examine their patients who are having gastrointestinal complaints including constipation or diarrhea. Have students document their findings and discuss their implications and possible nursing interventions.

3. In conference discuss how to adapt the abdominal exam when the patient has pain. Discuss pain assessment. When possible, relate to current patient situations.

TEST QUESTIONS

1. A positive Cullen's sign may indicate:
   A. appendicitis
 • B. intra-abdominal bleeding
   C. abdominal aortic aneurysm
   D. peritonitis

2. Percussion and palpation of the abdomen should be limited if:
   A. the patient has ascites
   B. bowel sounds are absent
 • C. an abdominal bruit is heard
   D. all of the above

3. Which of the following is true regarding rebound tenderness:
   A. it is a normal finding
   B. it is usually due to inflammation of the abdominal muscles
   C. it is frequently present with bowel obstruction
 • D. it may indicate peritonitis

4. A tympanic sound can be heard over:
   A. the liver
 • B. the stomach
   C. a stool filled colon
   D. bone

5. Which of the following allows for direct visualization of the common bile duct:
 • A. endoscopic retrograde cholangiopancre-atography (ERCP)
   B. colonoscopy
   C. decubitus films
   D. a barium study

6. Upper gastrointestinal endoscopy can be used to:
   A. visualize colon polyps
   B. determine the presence of free air in the abdominal cavity
 • C. sclerose esophageal varices
   D. evaluate the ileum

7. Which of the following studies is non-invasive:
   A. barium contrast studies
   B. colonoscopy
   C. paracentesis
 • D. ultrasonography

8. You are caring for a patient scheduled for an upper gastrointestinal endoscopy the next day. You would inform the patient:
   A. about the importance of a low-residue diet prior to the study
   B. how to administer enemas the evening prior to the study
   • C. to withhold oral intake for at least 8 hours prior to the study
   D. that he will be receiving an injection of contrast media prior to the study

9. Laxatives are most likely to be necessary following:
   A. abdominal ultrasonography
   • B. a barium swallow
   C. three-way abdominal films
   D. magnetic resonance imaging

10. Following his endoscopy, Mr. S. has begun complaining of severe shoulder and abdominal pain. His symptoms may be due to:
    • A. perforation, allowing air into the abdominal cavity
    B. a reaction to the contrast media

C. internal bleeding
D. the study itself; these are normal findings

11. Which of the following signs and symptoms are characteristic of an allergic reaction to contrast:
    A. fever, chills, hyperbilirubinemia
    B. hematemesis, tachycardia, hypotension
    • C. wheezing, hypotension
    D. adbominal pain that increases with movement

12. The patient should be observed for signs and symptoms of internal bleeding following:
    A. magnetic resonance imaging
    B. abdominal ultrasound
    • C. paracentesis
    D. computed axial tomography (CT)

13. A patient is admitted to rule out gallstones. Which study would you expect to be ordered:
    A. a radionuclide scan
    B. a barium swallow
    C. a colonoscopy
    • D. ultrasonography

CHAPTER 35

Management Modalities: Gastrointestinal System

BEHAVIORAL OBJECTIVES

Based on the content in this chapter, the reader should be able to:

1. Describe the body's metabolic response to a traumatic event.

2. State three parameters used to assess nutritional status.

3. Describe appropriate measures for

treatment of malnutrition.

4. State two complications of enteral hyperalimentation and two complications of central hyperalimentation.

5. Identify three nursing interventions for a patient receiving enteral hyperalimentation.

6. Identify three nursing interventions for a patient receiving central hyperalimentation.

OVERVIEW

Chapter 35 focuses on the nutritional assessment and support of critically ill patients. The body's metabolic response to illness and injury is explored and the physiological processes are examined in relation to catabolism and malnutrition. Nutritional assessment is described including a dietary history, anthropometric measurements, measurement of visceral proteins, and immunity and nitrogen balance studies. Factors which affect the patient's nutrition requirements are also explained.

Methods of nutritional support are described. The content on central hyperalimentation (TPN) examines the types of solutions, rate and volume of administration, the risk of infection, glucose intolerance, hepatic dysfunction and respiratory distress.

KEY TERMS

basal metabolic rate	glucagon
resting metabolic rate	anthropometric measurements
lipolysis	visceral proteins
catecholamines	fat emulsions

TEACHING/CLINICAL STRATEGIES

1. Have students make nursing rounds for patients receiving TPN and share with fellow students the cause of the malnutrition, laboratory values energy requirements and TPN solutions.

2. Have students describe key areas to assess in order to evaluate a patient's nutritional needs.

3. Conduct a case conference about a malnourished critically ill patient who receives TPN (e.g., a patient with acute pancreatitis or fulminating liver disease).

4. Have clinical specialist lecture on key principles in assessing a critically ill patient's nutritional status and the point at which nutritional support must be provided.

5. Have students choose a critically ill patient they have cared for and form small groups in which they discuss each patients' nutritional status, their risk of malnutrition, weight, anthropometric measures, energy needs, factors limiting their ability to meet energy requirements.

TEST QUESTIONS

1. A patient with a negative nitrogen balance:
   A. is anabolic
   B. is building protein from nitrogen supplies
 • C. is breaking down protein for use as energy
   D. is well nourished

2. The secretion of catecholamines in response to stress can result in:
   A. retention of water and sodium
 • B. hyperglycemia
   C. hypokalemia
   D. hypovolemia

3. Which of the following occurs during a catabolic state:
   A. uptake of glucose in peripheral tissues is increased
   B. insulin release is increased
   C. catecholamine secretion is supressed
   • D. glucagon is released

4. Which of the following is most likely to be seen in states of malnutrition:
   A. increased serum albumin levels
   B. positive nitrogen balance
   • C. decreased response to skin tests
   D. all of the above

5. Which of the following actions can help prevent diarrhea associated with enteral feedings:
   A. increasing the rate of the feeding
   B. decreasing the amount of water being added to the feedings
   C. administering the feeding as a bolus every 4 hours
   • D. changing the administration set every day

6. Your patient is receiving continuous full strength tube feedings at 100 cc/hour. The aspirated residual is 60 cc. The best action to take would be to:
   • A. hold the feeding for an hour and recheck the residual
   B. decrease the rate to 50 cc/hour
   C. change the concentration to one half strength
   D. lower the head of the bed until the residual is less than 20 cc

7. Which of the following is true regarding peripheral parenteral nutrition:
   A. it must be administered through a central venous catheter
   B. a 20% dextrose solution is commonly used
   C. lipids cannot be given peripherally
   • D. it is useful for short-term nutritional support

8. Mr. K. has become septic following a perforated diverticulum. In order to meet his nutritional needs, he should receive:
   A. a low residue diet with high protein and calorie supplements
   B. intermittant enteral feedings
   C. continous enteral feedings
   • D. total parenteral nutrition (TPN)

9. A common complication of peripheral parenteral nutrition is:
   • A. phlebitis
   B. aspiration
   C. osmotic diarrhea
   D. nausea and vomiting

10. Which of the following can the pharmacist add directly to the TPN solution:
    A. insulin
    B. potassium
    C. lipids
    • D. all of the above

11. Mrs. S. is receiving TPN at 100 cc/hour. Upon return from the radiology department, her nurse notices that the infusion pump is off and the TPN is now 200 cc behind schedule. The nurse should:
    A. restart the the infusion at 150 cc/hour in order to make up the lost volume
    • B. check the patients blood glucose level
    C. bolus the patient with 200 cc and then restart the infusion at 100 cc/hour
    D. administer a 5% dextrose solution

12. As you start your shift, you find that Mr. N.'s TPN is empty and the next bag is not ready yet. You should:
    A. cap his central venous catheter until the next bag of TPN is available
    • B. administer a 5% dextrose solution until the TPN is available
    C. administer a 0.9% saline solution until the TPN is available
    D. administer an extra dose of insulin to prevent rebound hyperglycemia

13. Which of the following is an appropriate nursing action when caring for a patient receiving TPN:
    A. change the tubing every other day
    B. add potassium to the currently infusing TPN solution when the patient becomes hypokalemic
    • C. monitor the patient's blood glucose levels
    D. all of the above

14. Mr. T. is receiving TPN through a single lumen central venous catheter. The physician has just ordered a unit of blood for Mr. T. Since he does not have another intravenous line in place the nurse should:
    A. piggyback the blood into the TPN tubing at the port closest to the patient
    B. stop the TPN and infuse the blood
    C. wait until this bag of TPN is finished, then infuse the blood before hanging the next TPN bag
    • D. start another intravenous line for the blood transfusion

165

CHAPTER 36

Acute Gastrointestinal Bleeding

Study Questions

BEHAVIORAL OBJECTIVES

Based on the content in this chapter, the reader should be able to:

1. Describe presenting signs and symptoms of acute gastrointestinal bleeding.

2. Identify the four steps in management of a patient with a gastrointestinal bleed.

3. Describe two treatments to control upper gastrointestinal bleeding.

4. Identify five nursing diagnoses and related nursing interventions for a patient experiencing an upper gastrointestinal bleed.

5. Describe the nursing management of a patient with a Sengstaken- Blakemore tube.

OVERVIEW

Chapter 36 presents content on acute gastrointestinal bleeding. The pathophysiology of bleeding from gastric and stress ulcers, and varices from chronic cirrhotic liver failure is discussed along with the history and clinical manifestations. Hematemesis, melena and other symptoms of bleeding are described as well as how to assess the severity of the blood loss. Laboratory values and their significance are discussed. Collaborative management focuses on counteracting shock by replacing fluids and blood products, diagnosing the cause; and planning and implementing treatment. Fluid replacement, gastric lavage, correcting clotting factor deficiencies and use of the balloon tamponade are examined. A case study and care plan are included.

KEY TERMS

hematemesis	hypocoagulable
melena	balloon tamponade
gastric lavage	vagotomy
sclerotherapy	antrectomy
histamine H2 antagonistic drugs	Billroth I and II

TEACHING/CLINICAL STRATEGIES

1. Arrange for student(s) to care for patients with acute GI bleeding.

2. In conference have students discuss hypovolemia and fluid replacement and compare and contrast pathophysiology, findings, assessment and management among patients with different medical diagnoses or injuries who also have hypovolemia and fluid replacement.

3. Using the case study and care plan in Chapter 36 discuss the patient's progress and nursing management during conference.

4. Arrange for student(s) to attend grand rounds for the GI service. In conference have student(s) share patients' findings and management.

TEST QUESTIONS

1. Upper gastrointestinal bleeding is most often caused by:
   A. esophageal varices
   - B. peptic ulcer disease
   C. ulcerative colitis
   D. malignant tumors

2. A history of coffee ground emesis indicates that the blood:
   A. is originating from the colon
   B. must be originating in the stomach
   - C. has been in contact with gastric secretions
   D. is originating below the ligament of Treitz

3. Which of the following signs or symptoms are most likely to be evidenced by the patient with a significant gastrointestinal bleed:
   - A. elevated blood urea nitrogen (BUN)
   B. absent bowel sounds
   C. rigid and hard abdomen
   D. all of the above

4. Gastric lavage has been ordered for Mrs. G. Which of the following solutions should the nurse instill into the patient's nasogastric tube:
   A. vasopressin
   B. iced normal saline
   - C. room temperature normal saline
   D. any of the above

5. Vasopressin may be used to manage gastrointestinal bleeding because it:
   A. decreases acid production by inhibiting histamine
   - B. decreases portal blood pressure
   C. causes sclerosis at the site of the bleed
   D. neutralizes gastric pH

6. When administering vasopressin, the nurse should monitor the patient for development of:
   A. respiratory insufficiency
   - B. hypertension
   C. dehydration due to excessive diuresis
   D. aspiration of gastric contents

7. Which of the following medications acts locally to protect the gastrointestinal mucosa:
   A. ranitidine hydrochloride
   B. levarterenol
   C. famotidine
   • D. sucralfate

8. Mr. K. has been receiving multiple antibiotics for treatment of pneumonia. He is endotracheally intubated and has been NPO and on intravenous feedings for 2 weeks. Now he has developed gastrointestinal bleeding. Which of the follwing could be the most likely cause:
   A. esophageal varices
   • B. vitamin K deficiency
   C. liver failure
   D. Mallory-Weiss tear

9. An appropriate action when placing a Sengstaken-Blakemore tube is:
   A. to inflate the gastric balloon with 100 cc of air then obtain a radiograph to check placement
   B. inflate the esophageal balloon with 50 cc of air for 24-48 hours
   • C. inflate the esophageal balloon to a pressure of 25-40 mm HG
   D. keep the gastric balloon deflated while the esophageal balloon is inflated

10. You are caring for Mrs. B., who has bleeding esophageal varices being managed with a Sengstaken-Blakemore tube. She suddenly seems to be having difficulty breathing. You should immediately:
    A. deflate the gastric balloon
    • B. cut and remove the tube
    C. increase the amount of pressure in the esophageal balloon
    D. increase the amount of traction on the tube

11. Inflation of the esophageal balloon for prolonged periods can cause:
    A. liver failure
    B. hypertension
    • C. esophagitis
    D. a Mallory-Weiss tear

12. The patient with liver failure and a gastrointestinal bleed is at increased risk of:
    • A. hepatic encephalopathy
    B. ascites formation
    C. hepatitis
    D. mesenteric infarction

13. An antrectomy:
    A. involves anastomosis of the stomach to the jejunum
    B. decreases parasympathetic stimulation to the stomach
    • C. removes acid producing cells in the stomach
    D. all of the above

14. A portal caval shunt diverts blood from:
    A. the vena cava into the portal vein
    B. the portal vein into the hepatic artery
    • C. the portal vein into the vena cava
    D. the hepatic artery into the vena cava

CHAPTER **37**

Hepatic Disorders

BEHAVIORAL OBJECTIVES

Based on the content in this chapter, the reader should be able to:

1. Identify four types of hepatitis.

2. Describe two liver disorders and their respective systems.

3. Identify five nursing diagnoses for the patient with liver failure.

4. Identify five nursing interventions for each nursing diagnosis.

OVERVIEW

Chapter 37 covers hepatitis and alcoholic cirrhosis of the liver accompanied by hepatic failure. The section on hepatitis describes five types: A, B, non A non B (C), D and drug induced. The incubation and contagious periods, symptoms, diagnosis and clinical course are described. Management encompasses providing rest and adequate nutrition.

Alcoholic cirrhosis of the liver explains the pathophysiological changes in the liver and porta system. Portal hypertension, altered metabolism, the inability to synthesize clotting factors and detoxify substances and the multisystem effects are described. Management examines the goals of supporting cardiopulmonary, hematological and nutritional functions of the liver, as well as, fluid balance. The effects of ascites and measures to relieve it are presented along with the complications of encephalopathy and hepatorenal syndrome. A nursing care plan on liver failure is included.

KEY TERMS

Kupffer's cells   IgM class antibodies

IgC class antibodies

TEACHING/CLINICAL STRATEGIES

1. Have student(s) care for patient(s) with hepatic failure and discuss their experiences in conference.

2. Conduct class on the complications of chronic cirrhosis of the liver including the pathophysiology, multisystem effects and nursing interventions.

3. Have students describe how they carry out precautions for blood borne pathogens.

TEST QUESTIONS

1. Which of the following is true regarding hepatits A:
   A. it can be spread by needle-stick injuries
   B. it frequently leads to chronic hepatitis
   • C. it is transmitted by the fecal-oral route
   D. it is the leading cause of fulminant liver failure

2. Management of hepatitis includes:
   A. a high protein, low carbohydrate diet
   • B. frequent rest periods
   C. administration of hepatitis B vaccine
   D. all of the above

3. Liver failure can result in:
   • A. hypoglycemia
   B. elevated serum albumin
   C. decreased serum ammonia levels
   D. hypermagnesemia

4. Mr. L. has been admitted with alcoholic cirrhosis of the liver. His family states that he has been increasingly confused, delirious, and agitated. Which of the following treatments is aimed at preventing further neurological changes:
   A. fluid restriction and diuretic therapy
   B. administration of fresh frozen plasma
   C. a high protein diet
   • D. administration of neomycin

5. You are caring for a patient with liver failure. Her laboratory studies reveal: blood urea nitrogen (BUN) = 45 mg/dl; serum creatinine = 3.0 mg/dl; albumin = 2.5 gm/dl. You suspect this is due to:
   A. low protein diet
   • B. hepatorenal syndrome
   C. diuretic therapy
   D. ascites

6. A direct complication of ascites is:
   A. hepatic encephalopathy
   B. hypertension
   • C. pleural effusion
   D. disseminated intravascular coagulation

7. Ascites can be managed by:
   A. administration of lactulose
   B. a low protein diet
   • C. fluid restriction
   D. all of the above

8. A Leveen shunt diverts:
   A. blood from the portal vein to the vena cava
   B. blood from the portal vein to the hepatic artery
   C. ascitic fluid from the peritoneum to the portal vein
   • D. ascitic fluid from the peritoneum to the vena cava

9. Which of the following can contribute to the development of hepatic encephalopathy:
   A. bleeding esophageal varices
   B. high protein diet
   C. presence of a portal-caval shunt

170

- D. all of the above

10. Mr. L. has liver failure. He is receiving lactulose in order to:
    A. increase renal perfusion
- B. reduce serum ammonia levels
    C. improve nitrogen balance
    D. prevent bleeding from esophageal varices

11. Which of the following laboratory values are most characteristic of liver failure:
- A. serum albumin = 2.0 gm/dl; prothrombin time (PT) = 20 seconds; lactic dehydrogenase (LDH) = 850 units
    B. serum albumin = 4.5 gm/dl; PT = 20 seconds; LDH = 300 units
    C. serum albumin = 6.0 gm/dl; PT = 13 seconds; LDH = 1200 units
    D. serum albumin = 2.0 gm/dl; PT = 13 seconds; LDH = 400 units

12. Which of the following contributes to ascites development:
    A. altered carbohydrate metabolism
- B. altered protein metabolism
    C. decreased ability of liver to detoxify substances
    D. decreased ability of liver to metabolize bile

13. Neomycin per nasogastric tube has been ordered for your patient with liver failure. You know that this will:
    A. prevent the ascitic fluid from becoming infected
    B. alter intestinal pH and increase ammonia excretion
- C. decrease the amount of bacteria in the colon
    D. cause osmotic diuresis and decrease ascites formation

CHAPTER **38**

Acute Pancreatitis

CHAPTER OUTLINE

Behavioral Objectives

Description

Pathophysiology

Assessment

  History

  Clinical Manifestations

  Diagnostic Studies

Management

  Fluid and Electrolyte Replacement

  Resting the Pancreas

  Pain Management

  Predicting Severity of Acute Pancreatitis

Complications

  Management of Systemic Complications

Case Study

Nursing Care Plan

Study Questions

BEHAVIORAL OBJECTIVES

Based on the content in this chapter, the reader should be able to:

1. Identify three major etiologies of acute pancreatitis.

2. Describe the pathophysiology of acute pancreatitis.

3. Name two presenting symptoms associated with acute pancreatitis.

4. List three diagnostic tests used to evaluate the patient for acute pancreatitis.

5. Name four major complications of acute pancreatitis.

6. Describe the multidisciplinary management of the patient with acute pancreatitis.

7. Develop a nursing care plan for the patient with acute pancreatitis.

OVERVIEW

Chapter 38 contains a concise overview of acute pancreatitis. It begins by explaining the causes and pathophysiology. This is followed by a discussion of the history and clinical findings along with the accompanying laboratory abnormalities and results of imaging tests which help diagnosis. Ranson's criteria, which help predict the severity of the disease, are included. Management examines fluid and electrolyte replacement, methods of resting the pancreas, pain management and complications. Concepts discussed in earlier chapters are applied and include hypovolemic shock, intake and output and hemodynamic monitoring. The significance of nothing by mouth and nasogastric tube drainage and the need for TPN are discussed as part of resting the pancreas. Principles of pain management and drugs of choice are covered. Enzyme release, hypovolemia and pancreatic abscesses and their multisystem complications are described. Peritoneal lavage and surgery to drain abscesses are also discussed. A case study and care plan are included.

KEY TERMS

alkaline phosphatase	retroperitoneal
autodigestive	pseudocyst
Grey Turner's sign	Mallory-Weiss
Cullen's sign	

TEACHING/CLINICAL SYNDROME

1. Have clinical specialist present a patient situation throughout the acute phase of care, highlighting history, cause, clinical findings, diagnostic and monitoring tools and nursing interventions.

2. Arrange for student(s) to participate in the care of a patient with acute pancreatitis and share their findings and interventions in conference.

3. Using the case study and care plan in Chapter 38, discuss the patient's course and accompanying interventions.

4. In class or conference have students research and then discuss pain control regimes for patients with acute pancreatitis and pain assessment tools; how to evaluate their effectiveness and how the regime can be changed. Invite a member of a hospital pain management team to participate.

5. In conference, have students discuss how the findings of an abdominal exam would be important in the patient's care, what they would look for and how they would conduct the exam for a patient with acute pancreatitis.

TEST QUESTIONS

1. An endocrine function of the pancreas is secretion of:
   - A. insulin
   - B. trypsin
   - C. aldosterone
   - D. elastase

2. Pancreatitis is caused by which of the following mechanisms:
   - A. endotoxins from the bowel causing inflammation of the pancreas
   - B. autodigestion by pancreatic enzymes
   - C. inability of the pancreas to activate it's enzymes
   - D. destruction of pancreatic tissue by bile

3. The signs and symptoms of acute pancreatitis will most likely include:
   - A. hyperactive bowel sounds, severe abdominal pain
   - B. steatorrhea, elevated blood urea nitrogen
   - C. vomiting, elevated serum amylase
   - D. decreased serum lipase, fever

4. When assessing a patient with acute pancreatitis, you elicit a positive Chvostek's sign. This most likely indicates:
   - A. hypokalemia
   - B. pleural effusion
   - C. hemorrhagic pancreatitis
   - D. hypocalcemia

5. Initial managment of pancreatitis includes:
   - A. diuretics
   - B. intravenous insulin
   - C. fluid replacement
   - D. calcium channel blockers

6. The analgesic of choice in managing pancreatic pain is:
   - A. morphine sulfate
   - B. demerol
   - C. aspirin
   - D. pain medication is contraindicated

7. Pancreatic secretions can be minimized by:
   A. inserting a nasogastric tube
   B. maintaining bed rest
   C. administering analgesics
 • D. all of the above

8. Mrs. P. has been admitted with pancreatitis. She is complaining of nausea, vomiting, and severe muscle weakness. Her electrocardiogram shows frequent premature ventricular contractions. Her symptoms are most likely due to:
   A. hyperglycemia
 • B. hypokalemia
   C. hypercalcemia
   D. hyponatremia

9. Which of the following can be a complication of acute pancreatitis:
   A. dysrhthmias, decreased cardiac output
   B. disseminated intravascular coagulation
   C. atelectasis, pleural effusion
 • D. all of the above

10. Mr. T. was admitted two weeks ago for acute pancreatitis. This is his second episode of pancreatitis and he is complaining of persistent nausea, vomiting, and abdominal pain. His temperature and serum amylase continue to be elevated. He may have developed:
 • A. a pancreatic pseudocyst

   B. disseminated intravascular coagulation
   C. peritonitis
   D. liver failure

11. Your patient is suffering from prolonged pancreatitis with complications. Her diet should include:
   A. clear liquids only
 • B. total parenteral nutrition without lipids
   C. foods low in fat
   D. enteral feedings

12. Mr. L. has been admitted with acute pancreatitis. He is receiving Ringer's lactate at 500 cc/hour. His blood pressure is 80/40 mm HG, pulmonary capillary wedge pressure = 6 mm HG, urine output = 15 cc in the last hour. He may benefit most from:
   A. diuretics
   B. changing to a normal saline solution
 • C. dopamine
   D. calcium channel blockers

13. Which of the following serum levels is most likely to be elevated in acute pancreatitis:
   A. calcium
   B. magnesium
   C. potassium
 • D. glucose

CHAPTER **39**

Anatomy and Physiology of the Endocrine System

175

BEHAVIORAL OBJECTIVES

Based on the content in this chapter, the reader should be able to:

1. Describe the production, actions, and regulation of ADH, growth and thyroid hormones, insulin and glucagon.

2. Identify how activated vitamin D, parathormone, and calcitonin each influence calcium metabolism.

3. Explain how glucocorticoids are secreted.

4. Summarize the renin-angiotensin mechanism for regulating mineralocorticoid secretion.

5. List 3 effects of pharmacological dosages of glucocorticoid medications.

6. Describe the site of manufacture, stimulus for secretion and action(s) of natriuretic hormone and erythropoietin.

OVERVIEW

Chapter 39 examines the structure and function of the major endocrine glands as well as natriuretic, erythropoietin and hormones which influence calcium metabolism. The focus is to provide a basis for pathophysiological crisis situations relevant to critical care nursing.

The manufacture, secretion, metabolic site, actions and regulations are discussed with emphasis on the communication role of endocrine secretions and their multisystem influences. Because of the far reaching and integrating effects of the endocrine system, this chapter will enhance understanding of this and other sections in the book. A table summarizes the site and actions of endocrine secretions.

KEY TERMS

cyclic AMP	optic chiasma
B receptors	paraventricular

B endorphin

pro-opiomelanocortin (POMC)

sympathetic-adrenal medulla (SAM) response

corticosteroid-binding globulin (CBG)

TEACHING/CLINICAL STRATEGIES

1. In conference have students apply knowledge of the physiology of endocrine secretions when caring for patients with endocrine related illness.

2. Have students describe the role of endocrine secretions when caring for patients with renal failure, fluid imbalance, burns, trauma, and cardiovascular crises.

TEST QUESTIONS

1. Which of the following hormones is released by the posterior pituitary gland:
   A. growth hormone
   B. parathormone
   - C. antidiuretic hormone (ADH)
   D. glucagon

2. ADH is secreted in response to:
   A. a decrease in plasma osmolality
   - B. a decrease in blood volume
   C. a rise in arterial blood pressure
   D. all of the above

3. Trauma to the hypothalamus can cause:
   A. altered calcium metabolism
   - B. excessive water excretion
   C. altered mineralocorticoid secretion
   D. all of the above

4. Calcium metabolism will be affected most by a lesion in the:
   A. posterior pituitary
   B. head of the pancreas
   C. adrenal medulla

- D. parathyroid

5. Calcium levels are elevated in response to:
   A. calcitonin
   B. growth hormone
   - C. parathormone
   D. all of the above

6. Glucose levels will rise in response to:
   - A. stimulation of alpha cells of the islets of langerhans
   B. stimulation of beta cells of the islets of langerhans
   C. supression of the adrenal medulla
   D. mineralocorticoids

7. Excessive ingestion of salt and water can lead to increased secretion of:
   A. erythropoietin
   B. renin
   C. aldosterone
   - D. natriuretic hormone

8. Excessive levels of which hormones can inhibit the inflammatory response:
   A. mineralocorticoids
   - B. glucocorticoids
   C. parathormone
   D. thyroid hormones

9. A patient presenting with tachycardia, hyperreflexia, weight loss, and diaphoresis most likely has:
   A. hypoparathyroidism
   B. a deficiency of mineralocorticoids
   C. pancreatic disease
   - D. hyperthyroidism

10. Surgical removal of the parathyroid glands would interfear with:
    A. production of red blood cells
    - B. calcium regulation
    C. temperature regulation
    D. glucose metabolism

11. Stimulation of beta islet cells results in:
    A. increased gluconeogenesis
    - B. increased glucose uptake by tissues

C. increased hepatic ketone production

D. increased glycogenolysis

12. Stress can cause:
    A. glucagon secretion
    B. stimulation of the adrenal medulla
    C. water retention
  • D. all of the above

13. Which of the following will cause extracellular fluid volume (ECF) to decrease:
    A. ADH
    B. renin
    C. aldosterone
  • D. natriuretic hormone

CHAPTER **40**

Diabetic Emergencies

BEHAVIORAL OBJECTIVES

Based on the content in this chapter, the reader should be able to:

1. Identify the two basic nutritional tasks of feeding and fasting.

2. Describe the brain's dependence on glucose.

3. Discuss the metabolic and hormonal activity that occurs in the four phases of nutrition - fed state, postabsorptive state, short fasting state, and prolonged fasting state.

4. Differentiate the two forms of diabetes - type I or insulin dependent diabetes (IDOM) and type II or non insulin dependent diabetes (NIDOM).

5. Identify the precipitating factors of diabetic ketoacidosis.

6. Describe the three major physiological disturbances of diabetic ketoacidosis - hyperosmolality, metabolic acidosis, and volume depletion.

7. Identify the clinical manifestations of diabetic ketoacidosis and concomittant complications.

8. Demonstrate knowledge of the principles underlying biochemical therapy for diabetic ketoacidosis - volume replacement, potassium and phosphorus replacement, and bicarbonate replacement.

9. Using a nursing diagnosis format, formulate a nursing care plan for patients with diabetic ketoacidosis.

10. Differentiate between the major physiological disturbances of diabetic ketoacidosis and hyperosmolar, hyperglycemic non ketotic coma.

11. Describe the neurological responses to a hypoglycemic episode.

OVERVIEW

Chapter 40 presents the diabetic emergencies of diabetic ketoacidosis, hyperosmolar hyperglycemic nonketotic coma and hypoglycemia. It should be read by all nursing students because the content includes principles which can be applied to any phase of diabetic care.

Because diabetes is a disease of disoriented nutrition, the physiological phases of feeding and fasting and the dependence of the brain on glucose for energy are examined along with the effects of uncontrolled diabetes on these physiological activities.

The section on diabetic ketoacidosis describes the pathophysiology, and clinical and diagnostic findings associated with hyperglycemia and hyperosmolality, ketosis and acidosis, and fluid and electrolyte losses. Management focuses on correcting these imbalances and includes salt and water replacement, correcting the acidosis, insulin replacement, and teaching sick day rules and other self management content in order to prevent reoccurrence.

The next section discusses hyperosmolar hyperglycemic nonketotic coma, the complication seen in older age type II diabetics. The history, clinical findings and management are described and these are compared and contrasted with diabetic ketoacidosis.

The last section explains hypoglycemia from the physiological perspective of the brain's dependence on glucose for energy. The history focuses on searching for cures since only then can patients be informed of ways to correct their self management. Clinical manifestations, diagnosis and management are discussed.

A case study and a care plan for diabetic ketoacidosis are included.

KEY TERMS

anticatabolic state	ketonuria
ketone bodies	Kussmaul breathing
glucagon	nitroprusside reagent
gluconeogenesis	osmotic diuresis
ketogenesis	

TEACHING/CLINICAL STRATEGIES

1. Conduct class on diabetic ketoacidosis and hyperosmolar hyperglycemic nonketotic coma, and hypoglycemia.

2. Have student(s) care for patient(s) with DK, HHNC, or hypoglycemia.

3. Have students review the record of a patient they have cared for and, in conference, discuss the symptoms, laboratory and clinical findings, management, the patient(s) version of what went wrong, and how it might be prevented in the future.

4. Using the case study and care plan (for Mr. Oliver) from Chapter 40, have students explain the pathophysiological events and the basis for the nursing interventions throughout the clinical course.

5. Have students develop a teaching plan based on the case study and care plan for Mr. Oliver.

TEST QUESTIONS

1. Glycogenolysis refers to:
   A. the storage of excess glucose in the liver
   B. the conversion of amino acids into glucose
   • C. the breakdown of glycogen by the liver
   D. the consumption of glucose by the brain

2. Which of the following nutrients provides an essential energy source for the brain:
   A. free fatty acids
   • B. glucose
   C. amino acids
   D. triglycerides

3. Which of the following hormones stimulates the storage of nutrients:
   • A. insulin
   B. glucagon
   C. growth hormone
   D. cortisol

4. The patient with diabetic ketoacidosis (DKA) will most likely exhibit:
   A. respiratory alkalosis
   B. respiratory acidosis
   C. metabolic alkalosis
   • D. metabolic acidosis

5. Volume depletion in the patient with DKA is a direct result of:
   - A. glycosuria
   - B. acidosis
   - C. decreased glomerular filtration
   - D. the brain's response to glucose deprivation

6. A 14 year old boy is admitted with DKA. He is exhibiting Kussmaul breathing. This is most likely:
   - A. a sign of respiratory acidosis
   - B. an attempt to compensate for metabolic acidosis
   - C. caused by central nervous system failure
   - D. a sign of underlying pneumonia

7. Ms. A. has a serum glucose of 800 mg/dl and her urine is positive for ketones. Which of the following would you also expect to see:
   - A. large urine output
   - B. decreased serum osmolality
   - C. metabolic alkalosis
   - D. elevated central venous pressure

8. Your patient has a serum glucose of 650 mg/dl. His potassium = 5.0 mEq/L, phosphate = 3.0 mg/dl, arterial pH = 7.25. As treatment is begun with intravenous normal saline and low dose insulin the patient may develop:
   - A. hyperphosphatemia
   - B. hypokalemia
   - C. worsening acidosis
   - D. all of the above

9. Which of the following is most characteristic of the patient with hyperosmolar hyperglycemic nonketotic coma:
   - A. type I diabetes; serum glucose = 800 mg/dl; potassium = 6.0 mEq/L
   - B. type II diabetes; serum glucose = 600 mg/dl; anion gap = 20 mEq/L
   - C. 25 years old; serum glucose = 1000 mg/dl; sodium = 132 mEq/L
   - D. 65 years old; serum glucose = 1200 mg/dl; anion gap = 6 mEq/L

10. In comparison with hyperosmolar hyperglycemic nonketotic coma, the patient with DKA usually presents with a higher:
    - A. serum glucose
    - B. serum sodium
    - C. anion gap
    - D. serum osmolality

11. Treatment of hyperosmolar hyperglycemic nonketotic coma should begin with:
    - A. fluid replacement
    - B. high doses of insulin
    - C. bicarbonate administration
    - D. potassium administration

12. A 20 year old with type I diabetes has just been admitted. He is very lethargic and stuporous. His respirations are rapid and deep, heart rate is elevated, and he is hypotensive. His friends say that he has been vomiting the last few days. He is most likely suffering from:
    - A. DKA
    - B. hyperosmolar hyperglycemic nonketotic coma
    - C. insulin reaction
    - D. somogyi effect

13. A 40 year old insulin dependent diabetic is becoming increasingly stuporous. He is pale, diaphoretic, and tachycardic. The initial treatment of choice in this case is:
    - A. a low dose insulin infusion
    - B. a bolus of high dose insulin
    - C. a bolus of 50% dextrose
    - D. fluid replacement

14. An insulin dependent patient suffering from gastroenteritis and vomiting should:
    - A. stop his insulin until he is able to eat again
    - B. take half his usual insulin dose while he is ill
    - C. monitor his blood glucose levels and use only long acting insulin if needed
    - D. monitor his blood glucose levels and take supplemental doses of short acting insulin if needed

15. Hyperosmolar hyperglycemic nonketotic coma differs from DKA in that:
- A. mortality and complication rates are higher
  B. it usually occurs in younger patients
  C. volume depletion is not as severe
  D. all of the above

CHAPTER **41**

Common Endocrine Disorders

BEHAVIORAL OBJECTIVES

Based on the content in this chapter, the reader should be able to:

1. Describe the pathophysiological principles of thyroid crises, myxedema coma, adrenal crises and SIADH.

2. Identify key precipitating factors, laboratory findings and clinical manifestations for each of these disorders.

3. Discuss nursing diagnosis and interventions for the acute phase of each of these disorders.

OVERVIEW

Chapter 41 covers four endocrine emergencies: thyroid and adrenal crises, myxedema coma and SIADH. The pathophysiology, precipitating causes, clinical findings, management, including drug treatment, and complications are described. Also included are risk factors for these disorders, subtle clinical parameters and the differing presentation in the elderly.

A nursing care plan for each disorder is included.

KEY TERMS

thyrotoxicosis   mucopolysaccharides

propylthiouracil

TEACHING/CLINICAL STRATEGIES

1. Invite an endocrinologist to lecture on the most common endocrine crises.

2. Arrange for student(s) to attend grand rounds on an endocrine unit and share some key points in conference.

3. In conference have students discuss the multisystem effects of thyroid and adrenal crises and nursing interventions.

4. In conference or class discuss the clinical findings, management and care plan for the patient with hyponatremia (Care Plan 23-1).

TEST QUESTIONS

1. Undiagnosed Grave's disease can lead to:
   * A. thyroid crisis
   B. myxedema coma
   C. adrenal crisis
   D. syndrome of inappropriate antidiuretic hormone secretion (SIADH)

2. Signs and symptoms of hyperthyroidism include:
   A. cool, clammy skin; bradycardia; hypothermia
   B. weight gain; decreased appetite; tachycardia
   * C. fever; agitation; palpitations
   D. hyperpigmentation; hyperkalemia; seizures

3. Propylthiouracil:
   A. increases levels of T3
   * B. blocks conversion of T4 to T3
   C. is used to manage symptoms of hypothyroidism
   D. is a synthetic form of T4

4. The use of beta-adrenergic blockers in the presence of hyperthyroidism:
   A. can exacerbate the cardiac signs and symptoms of hyperthyroidism
   B. is contraindicated
   * C. may mask the cardiac symptoms of thyroid crisis
   D. will inhibit thyroid hormone release

5. Mr. T. is complaining of fatigue, weakness, anorexia, and weight gain. His voice is hoarse and he has non-pitting edema of the hands and around his eyes. He is exhibiting signs and symptoms of:
   A. Addison's disease
   B. Grave's disease
   C. SIADH
   * D. hypothyroidism

6. Mrs. S. has been diagnosed with myxedema coma. Which of the following electrolyte imbalances would you expect her to have:
   A. hyperkalemia
   * B. hyponatremia
   C. hyperglycemia
   D. hypocalcemia

7. In addition to administration of thyroid hormone, management of myxedema coma may also include:
   A. mechanical ventilation
   B. vasopressors
   C. corticosteroids
   * D. all of the above

8. Complications of hypothyroidism include:
   * A. paralytic ileus
   B. malignant hypertension
   C. pulmonary edema
   D. all of the above

9. A patient with adrenal insufficiency will most likely have elevated levels of:
   A. glucose
   - B. potassium
   C. sodium
   D. bicarbonate

10. Mrs. B. presents with orthostatic hypotension, weight loss, hyponatremia, hyperkalemia, and an elevated blood urea nitrogen. She complains of vomiting, diarrhea, and abdominal pain. She is afebrile and her heart rate = 108/minute. Management of her condition will most likely begin with:
    A. hypertonic saline and furosemide
    B. demeclocycline
    C. propylthiouracil
    - D. hydrocortisone and fluid replacement

11. Mr. K. has oat cell carcinoma of the lung. He is currently admitted with acute mental status changes and a sodium of 118 mEq/L. His diagnosis most likely is:
    A. hypothyroidism
    B. Grave's disease
    - C. SIADH
    D. diabetes insipidus

12. Which of the following laboratory findings is consistent with SIADH:

A. blood urea nitrogen = 45 mg/dl
- B. serum osmolality = 250 mOsm
C. serum sodium = 145 mEq/L
D. urine specific gravity = 1.001

13. Fluid imbalances associated with SIADH may be managed with:
    A. hypotonic saline
    - B. fluid restriction
    C. colloids
    D. 5% dextrose

14. Mineralocorticoid deficiency can result in:
    A. hypoglycemia
    B. hypercalcemia
    - C. hyperkalemia
    D. hypernatremia

15. Mrs. L. is admitted following a seizure. She is hypothermic, bradycardic, and hypotensive. She also exhibits periorbital edema. Which of the following laboratory findings would you expect:
    - A. decreased T4 levels
    B. decreased serum cortisol levels
    C. hyperkalemia
    D. decreased serum osmolality

CHAPTER 42

Septic Shock

CHAPTER OUTLINE

BEHAVIORAL OBJECTIVES

Based on the content in this chapter, the reader should be able to:

1. Define septic shock.

2. Identify risk factors associated with the development of septic shock.

3. Describe the pathophysiologic processes implicated in septic shock.

4. Explain the anticipated medical management and rationale for the treatment of septic shock.

5. Identify four nursing diagnoses and interventions for the patient in septic shock.

OVERVIEW

Chapter 42 examines septic shock which occurs frequently and is often fatal. The cause, risk factors and pathophysiology are discussed. Multisystem clinical manifestations are covered beginning with decreased and poorly distributed circulation. Poor cardiac function due to lactic acidosis, respiratory problems, coagulopathy, and widespread metabolic disturbances are examined. Management integrates concepts presented in other units and includes treating the infection, restoring intravascular volume, and maintaining adequate cardiac output, ventilation, metabolism, and nutrition. A case study and care plan are included.

KEY TERMS

endotoxin	hyperdynamic shock
exotoxin	hypodynamic shock
systemic vascular resistance (SVR)	kreb's cycle
lactic acidemia	

TEACHING/CLINICAL STRATEGIES

1. Invite clinical specialist to discuss nursing interventions surrounding the multisystem assessment of septic shock.

2. In conference discuss the case study about Mrs. Cox. Have students review her clinical course and compare laboratory values, clinical signs and symptoms; and discuss pathophysiological events and nursing interventions.

   a) Discuss the dose, actions and desired outcomes of the dopamine and dobutamine given to Mrs. Cox.

   b) Have students discuss how they would adapt the abdominal exam for Mrs. Cox and what they might expect to find.

   c) Have students set up a plan for weaning Mrs. Cox from the ventilator. (Have students refer to Chapter 19.) Discuss assessing her physiological and psychosocial readiness using adaptation to illness concepts from Chapter 2.

TEST QUESTIONS

1. Septic shock is frequently the result of an inflammatory response caused by:
   A. gram negative endotoxin
   B. gram positive exotoxin
   C. viral infections
   • D. all of the above

2. The hemodynamic effects seen with septic shock are:
   A. hypotension, low SVR, low cardiac output
   • B. hypotension, low SVR, high cardiac output
   C. hypovolemia, hypotension, low cardiac output
   D. vasodilation, high SVR, high cardiac output

3. High urinary nitrogen excretion is evidence of:
   A. renal insufficiency
   B. hypovolemia
   • C. protein breakdown
   D. liver failure

4. The most important initial therapy for the patient in septic shock is:
   A. identify and treat the infection
   B. monitor urine output
   • C. restore intravascular volume
   D. assure adequate nutrition

5. J.L. is in septic shock, has ARDS, and is intubated and on a ventilator. His CO = 10.5 L/min, Pcw = 18 mmHg, SVR = 500 dynes/second/cm-5 and BP = 80/46 mmHg. The nurse would expect to:
   A. give more fluids
   B. administer Nipride
   • C. administer Dopamine
   D. restrict fluids

6. Potential drug therapies for septic shock include all but:
   A. monoclonal antibodies
   • B. tumor necrosis factor

C. antihistamines

D. steroids

7. Coagulation problems that develop in septic shock are the result of:
- A. complement activation
  B. clotting factor depletion
  C. factor deficiency
  D. excessive platelet production

8. The patient with hypotension, low cardiac output, high SVR and cool pale skin is manifesting signs of:
  A. the hyperdynamic phase of septic shock
  B. hypovolemic shock
- C. the hypodynamic phase of septic shock
  D. none of the above

9. In caring for the patient in multiple organ failure after septic shock, the nurse should:
- A. help the patient's family understand the poor prognosis associated with this situation
  B. remain optimistic for a full recovery
  C. educate the family about potential investigational therapies being used to treat sepsis
  D. all of the above

10. Patients at risk to develop sepsis include:
  A. immunosuppressed patients
  B. the very young and the very old
  C. patients without a spleen
- D. all of the above

CHAPTER 43

Disseminated Intravascular Coagulation

CHAPTER OUTLINE

Behavioral Objectives

Description

Physiological Principles

  Hemostatic System

    Intrinsic Pathway

    Extrinsic Pathway

  Coagulation Inhibitors

    Reticuloendothelial System

      Fibrinolytic System Inhibitors

Disseminated Intravascular Coagulation

  Pathophysiology

Assessment

  Clinical Manifestations

  Diagnostic Studies

Management

  Eliminate Cause

  Minimize Further Bleeding

  Replace Depleted Factor

  Heparin Therapy

  Antithrombin Iii Concentrate

Complications

  Related to Bleeding

  Related to Thrombosis

Case Study

Nursing Care Plan

Study Questions

BEHAVIORAL OBJECTIVES

Based on the content in this chapter, the reader should be able to:

1. Describe the pathophysiological process of disseminated intravascular coagulation (DIC).

2. List the abnormal laboratory findings associated with DIC.

3. Explain the anticipated medical management and rationale for the treatment of DIC.

4. Describe four nursing diagnoses and interventions for DIC.

OVERVIEW

Chapter 43 explains the physiological concepts of coagulation which include hemostatic factors and coagulation inhibitors and their role in maintaining equilibrium. The risk factors and pathophysiological events causing DIC are examined, along with the need for early recognition and treatment of those at risk. Early signs and symptoms are described along with abnormal laboratory data and possible multisystem problems. Management discusses eliminating the cause, minimizing further bleeding, correcting the clotting deficiency and treating complications resulting from bleeding or thrombosis.

KEY TERMS

hypercoagulable

extrinsic pathway

fibrinolytic

reticuloendothelial system

coagulation factors

intrinsic pathway

fibrinolytic system

TEACHING/CLINICAL STRATEGIES

1. Arrange for student(s) to care for patient(s) with DIC and then share their experience in conference.

2. Arrange for a nurse specialist to present nursing rounds or case situations of patients with DIC and discuss assessment and nursing interventions.

3. Have students discuss the case study RP in Chapter 44. Evaluate symptoms, laboratory data and management. Compare and contrast the assessment and management of DIC and septic shock.

TEST QUESTIONS

1. Platelets are involved in the clotting process in which of the following ways:
   - A. they form initial platelet plug at the site of the vessel tear
   B. they initiate the extrinsic pathway
   C. they activate plasminogen
   D. they convert prothrombin to thrombin

2. Mast cells, located in most body tissues, are involved in the inhibition of coagulation as they:
   A. produce plasminogen
   B. activate the reticuloendothelial system
   - C. produce heparin
   D. none of the above

3. The following lab values are increased with DIC:
   A. fibrinogen level
   - B. fibrin degredation products
   C. plasminogen levels
   D. platelet count

4. The triggering event in DIC causes:
   - A. systemic coagulation activity
   B. uncontrolled bleeding
   C. excessive platelet production
   D. activation of the fibrinolytic system

5. The mainstay of therapy in DIC is:
   A. blood replacement
   B. clotting factor replacement
   - C. elimination of the cause
   D. heparin therapy

6. The goal of heparin therapy is to:
   - A. stop the cycle of thrombosis
   B. dissolve existing clots
   C. activate thrombin
   D. promote platelet aggregation

7. The nurse is caring for a patient in hypovolemic shock secondary to multiple trauma. On physical exam the nurse notes small areas of petechiae on the arms of the patient. What other parameters should the nurse assess?
   A. guiac test stools
   B. nasogastric aspirant pH
   C. bleeding at puncture sites
   - D. all of the above

8. Altered mental status in a patient in DIC may be a sign of:
   A. hypoxemia
   - B. intracerebral bleeding
   C. head trauma
   D. electrolyte imbalance

9. Priorities in nursing care for the patient in DIC include:
   A. skin care
   B. avoid/limit injections or skin punctures
   C. critical evaluation of complaints of pain

- D. all of the above

10. Heparin therapy is used in DIC to:
- A. slow the coagulation process to promote restoration of coagulation proteins
  B. promote thrombin production
  C. promote platelet aggregation
  D. all of the above

CHAPTER **44**

Trauma

BEHAVIORAL OBJECTIVES

Based on the content in this chapter, the reader

should be able to:

1. Outline the four phases of initial assessment and care of the trauma patient.

2. Discuss the treatment of and nursing actions associated with trauma to the chest and heart.

3. Contrast the response of solid and hollow abdominal organs to trauma.

4. Describe management of and nursing actions related to abdominal trauma.

5. Identify two serious complications of pelvic trauma.

6. Describe the nursing responsibilities associated with trauma to the extremities.

7. List the disorders involved in multiple organ failure.

OVERVIEW

Chapter 44 presents the assessment, management and complications of trauma. Thoracic, abdominal, pelvic and extremity injuries are included. This chapter integrates content from all other units and gives the reader an opportunity to apply earlier learning to care of injured patients.

The four phases of initial hospital assessment and management are addressed: primary evaluation, resuscitation, secondary assessment and definitive care. Clues to recognizing early signs and symptoms of multiple injuries are described along with diagnostic findings and surgical interventions. Hemorrhage, head injury and multiple organ failure and their accompanying mortality rates are discussed. A case study and a care plan are included.

KEY TERMS

pneumatic antishock garment (PASG)

diagnostic peritoneal lavage (DPL)

perihepatic abscess

overwhelming postplenectomy sepsis (OPSS)

ankle brachial indexes (ABI's)

TEACHING/CLINICAL STRATEGIES

1. Arrange for clinical experience in emergency, trauma and critical care areas.

2. Invite a flight nurse and trauma team nurse to discuss the nursing responsibilities during the prehospital and initial phases of care.

3. In conference have a critical care specialist discuss the nursing responsibilities during the definitive phase of care.

4. In conference present the case study and care plan from Chapter 44 or a current patient situation. Have students discuss the predisposing factors, findings and nursing interventions for sepsis, ARDS and ARF.

5. Invite trauma team and CCU nurses to dialogue with students about factors that create job stress and their coping styles. Assign Chapter 10, Effects of the Critical Care Unit on the Nurse, as prereading and have students prepare questions for the panel of nurses.

TEST QUESTIONS

1. Which of the following must be performed during the primary evaluation at an accident scene:
   A. endotracheal intubation

- B. assessment of airway, breathing, and circulation
  C. a diagnostic peritoneal lavage
  D. a thorough medical history

2. Primary assessment of a motor vehicle accident (MVA) victim reveals: increasing respiratory distress, absent breath sounds over the upper third of the right lung, tachycardia, and probable fracture of the right humerus. Which of the following would be the best action for the nurse to take next:
   A. obtain an electrocardiogram
   B. inqure about medication allergies
   - C. prepare for insertion of a chest tube
   D. splint the fracture

3. Which of the following nursing actions is appropriate for the patient with a flail chest:
   - A. encouraging coughing and deep breathing
   B. taping the fractured ribs tightly
   C. withholding analgesics
   D. all of the above

4. Which of the following is characteristic of pulmonary contusion:
   A. sudden onset of respiratory failure
   - B. increasing peak airway pressures
   C. diffuse infiltrates seen on a chest radiograph
   D. usually associated with respiratory alkalosis

5. Managment of a patient with pulmonary contusion is most likely to include:
   A. strict fluid restriction
   B. high frequency jet ventilation
   C. insertion of chest tubes
   - D. mechanical ventilation with positive end-expiratory pressure (PEEP)

6. Mr. X. is admitted following a MVA. Upon assessment, the nurse discovers that he is tachycardic, hypotensive, has distended neck veins, and muffled heart sounds. The nurse suspects he has a:
   A. cardiac contusion

B. pneumothorax
- C. cardiac tamponade
  D. torn aortic arch

7. Immediately following surgery to repair a transected aorta, nursing care is most likely to include:
   A. strict fluid restriction
   - B. administration of a vasodilator
   C. mechanical ventilation with high levels of PEEP
   D. serial monitoring of cardiac enzyme levels

8. Mrs. L. underwent a splenorrhaphy two days ago, following a MVA. She also has fractures of her three lower left ribs. Now she is complaining of nausea, vomiting, and epigastric pain radiating to her back. Her hematocrit = 35%. Serum amylase is elevated. Which of the following may be causing her signs and symptoms:
   - A. undiagnosed pancreatic injury
   B. overwhelming post-splenectomy sepsis (OPSS)
   C. pneumonia
   D. associated renal injury

9. Following multiple stab wounds to the colon, Mr. P. is at an increased risk for the development of:
   A. malabsorption syndrome
   B. pancreatitis
   - C. intra-abdominal sepsis
   D. disseminated intravascular coagulation (DIC)

10. Mr. D. sustained severe liver lacerations in a motorcycle accident. Following segmental resection he continues to hemorrhage from the surgical site. The nurse anticipates that he will require:
    - A. further hepatic surgery
    B. an abdominal CT scan
    C. blood products to manage his newly developed DIC

D. application of a pneumatic anti-shock garment (PASG)

11. Following a severe pelvic fracture, the critical care nurse's primary goal is to:
    A. preserve range of motion and facilitate early ambulation
    B. assess for the development of peritonitis
    C. assess for the development of DIC
  • D. prevent hemorrhagic shock

12. Bladder injury should be suspected in the presence of:
    A. lower rib fractures
  • B. pelvic fractures
    C. renal injuries
    D. all of the above

13. Mr. K. suffered head injuries, right sided flail chest and pulmonary contusion, multiple hepatic lacerations, and fractures of the right humerus and right femur in a MVA. He is at risk of developing which of the following complications:
    A. adult respiratory distress syndrome (ARDS)
    B. DIC
    C. sepsis
  • D. all of the above

14. Which of the following patients is at risk of developing ARDS:
    A. the patient with sepsis following hepatic trauma
    B. the patient with bilateral pulmonary contusions
    C. the patient who received 45 units of blood following a pelvic fracture
  • D. all of the above

15. Which of the following is true regarding multiple organ failure (MOF):
    A. the first organ to fail is usually the heart
  • B. early nutritional support may decrease the development of MOF
    C. MOF occurs in 50% of critically injured patients
    D. all of the above

CHAPTER **45**

Burns

BEHAVIORAL OBJECTIVES

Based on the content in this chapter, the reader should be able to:

1. Use a burn classification system.

2. Describe the major pathophysiological changes associated with burn injury.

3. Describe the major psychological changes associated with burn injury.

4. Define the phases of recovery following burn injury.

5. Identify the major clinical problems in each phase of recovery following burn injury.

6. State the rationale for specific management of major clinical problems in each phase of recovery following burn injury.

7. Develop a nursing care plan for the patient in each phase of recovery following burn injury.

OVERVIEW

Chapter 45 presents a very thorough discussion of burns and is valuable reading for all nursing students. Content begins by exploring hypovolemic shock, a major pathophysiological result of burn injury. The depth, causes and severity of burns are described along with key points for the early identification of inhalation injury. The hematological response to burn injury is explained along with the electrolyte, metabolic and renal sequelae of burns.

Managing the burn injury is explored throughout the resuscitative, acute and rehabilitative phases. During the resuscitative phase, principles of fluid administration, as well as treatment of inhalation injury, tissue perfusion, wound care, pain and psychosocial support are covered. The acute phase focuses on managing the burn wound, preventing infection, would debridement, grafting and nutrition. The rehabilitative phase covers promoting nutrition, and avoiding scarring and contractures. There is a nursing care plan for each phase.

KEY TERMS

fluid resuscitation	full thickness
debridement	biological dressing
escharotomy	non protein
superficial partial thickness	collagens
deep partial thickness	split thickness grafts

TEACHING/CLINICAL STRATEGIES

1. Arrange for a clinical specialist to present a case situation which illustrates the assessment and management concepts during the resuscitative and acute phases. Also include rehabilitative measures which are started in CCU.

2. Arrange for student(s) to participate in rounds on a burn unit and share key points in clinical conference.

3. Arrange for student(s) to participate in the care of a burn patient and share the major nursing diagnosis and interventions.

4. Have student(s) obtain data regarding the major causes of fires and then develop a risk profile and assessment tool. Also have them review the fire procedures at their residence and clinical sites.

5. Provide a patient situation which describes a burn injury. Using the rule of nine and initial fluid replacement principles, have students estimate the extent of the burn, the risk for inhalation injury and the amount of fluid replacement needed the first 24 hours.

TEST QUESTIONS

1. Burn shock, a form of hypovolemic shock, is largely a process of:
   A. fluid shifts from the burn area into the vascular space
   B. fluid loss at the burn site
   - C. fluid shifts from the vascular space into the interstitial areas of the burn wound
   D. extensive bleeding secondary to debridement

2. A burn that involves the epidermis and dermal layers and is red, painful and edematous is classified as a:
   A. full thickness burn
   B. deep partial-thickness burn
   C. first degree burn
   D. third degree burn

3. C.J. was burned during a lab explosion. She has burns to her left arm, her left anterior leg, and the left anterior trunk. Using the rules of nine's, her calculated TBSA would be:
   A. 36%
   B. 18%
   C. 22.5%
   - D. 27%

4. Signs of a potential inhalation injury include:
   A. singed nasal hairs
   B. coughing up soot
   C. hoarse voice
   - D. all of the above

5. Treatment for suspected inhalation injury will include:
   A. immediate endotracheal intubation
   B. immediate tracheostomy
   - C. administration of humidified oxygen
   D. bronchoscopy and debridement of burned tissue

6. T.J. weighs 65 kg and has 35% TBSA burned. Using the Parkland formula, the amount of fluid necessary in the first 8 hrs would be:
   - A. 4,550 ml
   B. 9,100 ml
   C. 6,350 ml
   D. 2,150 ml

7. The fluid of choice for initial fluid replacement is:
   A. DSW
   B. .9 Normal Saline
   C. colloid
   - D. lacted ringers solution

8. A.D. has a 60% TBSA 2nd and 3rd degree burn. While monitoring intake and output, the nurse notes dark brown urine. This is probably the result of:
   A. hemoconcentration
   - B. myoglobin

C. melanin

D. alkalosis

9. K.L. has circumfrentrial burns to his arms. Upon assessment the nurse notes decreased capillary refill, pallor and numbness in the R hand. This most likely indicates:
- A. poor circulation and the need for esharatomy
  B. ischemia and the need for faciotomy
  C. thrombosis
  D. compartment syndrome

10. Most medications should be given intravenously during the resuscitative phase of burn management except:
  A. pain medications
  B. antibiotics

- C. tetanus toxoid
  D. none of the above

11. The best method to limit infection at burn sites is with the use of:
  A. sterile dressings and coverings
  B. sterile saline flushes
- C. topical antimicrobial agents
  D. all of the above

12. During the acute phase of burn management, priority nursing activities are aimed at:
  A. fluid volume replacement
- B. wound management
  C. airway maintenance
  D. preventing contractures

CHAPTER **46**

Drug Overdose and Poisoning

CHAPTER OUTLINE

BEHAVIORAL OBJECTIVES

Based on the content in this chapter, the reader
should be able to:

1. Discuss the initial assessment and
   management for acutely poisoned
   patients.

2. Describe the different methods to prevent
   absorption and enhance elimination in the
   management of the acutely poisoned
   patient.

3. Describe the groups of symptoms or
   toxidromes that may assist in identifying
   the drug(s) or toxin(s) to which the patient
   may have been exposed.

4. Develop a care plan for the poisoned
   patient.

OVERVIEW

Chapter 46 presents the prevalence of drug overdose and poisoning and important information about how to respond. The response to immediate and life threatening problems, and key points in history taking and identifying the toxin are describes. Management discusses five types of exposures to toxins and immediate ways to prevent further absorption. Measures to eliminate substances from the body are described and include the use of emetics, lavage, adsorbents, cathartics, hemodialysis and hyperbaric oxygenation therapy. A case study and care plan for the patient with cocaine toxicity is included.

KEY TERMS

toxidromes

gastrointestinal decontamination

adsorption

emetics

Syrup of Ipecac

activated charcoal

whole bowel irrigation

hemoperfusion

hyperbaric oxygenation therapy

antagonists

TEACHING/CLINICAL STRATEGIES

1. Arrange for a nurse or pharmacist from the area poison control center to present data on common poisonings and overdoses.

2. In conference have students discuss patients they have cared for who have had drug or toxin poisoning.

3. Have students each choose a substance from Table 46-5 and identify how people may become exposed, preventive measures and key points in assessment and management present briefly in class or conference.

4. Arrange for a nurse substance abuse counselor to discuss drug addiction and post crisis nursing interventions.

5. Have students discuss how to "child proof" a house for substances toxic to children.

TEST QUESTIONS

1. L.T. was found unresponsive at home with an empty bottle of Valium and gin nearby. The initial pharmacologic management should include:
   A. activated charcoal
   - B. dextrose, narcan, oxygen
   C. syrup of ipecac
   D. all of the above

2. Bradycardia, excessive salivation, pulmonary edema, pinpoint pupils may result from:
   A. narcotic overdose
   B. anticholinergic drugs
   C. cocaine overdose
   - D. organophosphate poisoning

3. Syrup of ipecac is contraindicated with:
   A. caustic ingestions
   B. absent gag reflex
   C. seizures
   - D. all of the above

4. During gastric lavage the patient should be:
   A. in the high fowlers position
   - B. in the left lateral decubitus position
   C. flat in bed
   D. prone with the head lower than the feet

5. Activated charcoal:
   A. will only absorb drug remaining in the GI system
   B. is contraindicated in patients with a depressed level of consciousness
   C. is effective in lithium overdose
   - D. none of the above

202

6. L.C. has ingested an overdose of Tylenol. The nurse will anticipate the following intervention:
   A. urine alkalinization
   B. activated charcoal and N-acetylcysteine administration
   - C. n-acetylcysteine administration
   D. hemodialysis

7. Hyperbaric oxygen therapy is indicated for:
   A. carbon monoxide poisoning
   B. methylene chloride inhalation
   - C. both A & B
   D. none of the above

8. J.K. has taken an intentional overdose of Nortriptyline. The nurse will need to closely assess his:
   - A. cardiac status, EKG

   B. hepatic function
   C. renal function
   D. all of the above

9. The antidote for ethylene glycol ingestion is:
   A. activated charcoal
   B. not yet available
   C. mucomyst
   - D. ethanol

10. Toxins that can cause an elevated anion gap include:
    A. windshield washer fluid
    B. antifreeze
    C. aspirin
    - D. all of the above

CHAPTER 47

Immune System Compromising Conditions

CHAPTER OUTLINE

BEHAVIORAL OBJECTIVES

Based on the content in this chapter, the reader should be able to:

1. Describe the physiology of adaptive immune responses.

2. Discuss the etiologies of impaired host defenses and resistance.

3. Outline appropriate nursing assessment parameters related to immunocompetence of the critically ill patient.

4. Describe the etiology, immunopathology, and medical and nursing interventions associated with acquired immunodeficiency syndrome (AIDS).

5. Discuss the incidence and development of nosocomial infections in the critically ill patient.

6. Explain universal precautions and their implementation in the critical care unit.

OVERVIEW

Chapter 47 discusses the assessment and management of the critically ill patient with AIDS. To enhance understanding of the issues facing immunocompromised patients, this chapter also examines principles of innate and adaptive immune responses. The latter includes a discussion of humoral and cell-mediated immunity. Assessment of the immunocompromised patient focuses on seven areas including nutritional status, skin integrity and medications. The section on AIDS encompasses the transmission, immune defects and the clinical manifestation and management of respiratory and central nervous system opportunistic infections. The last section describes nosocomial infections and the steps necessary to reduce their incidence. A case study and care plan for the patient with AIDS is included.

KEY TERMS

innate immunity	cytoxic T cells
phagocytosis	helper/inducer T cells
adaptive immunity	
humoral immunity	suppressor T cells
cell-mediated immunity	delayed-type hypersensitivity cells
T lymphocytes	retroviruses

TEACHING/CLINICAL STRATEGIES

1. Arrange for students to care for patients who are seriously ill with opportunistic infections such as pneumocystis carinii pneumonia.

2. Using a current clinical situation or the case study and care plan in Chapter 47, have students discuss the clinical course and nursing interventions for a patient critically ill with PCP.

3. Using the case study in Chapter 47 have students discuss and then role play how they would talk with the family (including the S O) about their feelings now that Mr. J was not likely to survive and would not be resuscitated.

4. In conference have students discuss the measures they have taken that day to prevent transmitting infection to their patients.

5. Arrange a lecture on the latest drug management for AIDS and the major opportunistic infections

TEST QUESTIONS

1. The type of immunity that does not require a previous exposure to the organism or toxin is termed:
   A. adaptive immunity
   B. cell-mediated immunity
 • C. innate immunity
   D. humoral immunity

2. Neutrophils:
   A. are produced in the thymus
 • B. provide the "first wave" of attack in the inflammatory process
   C. are fewer in number than monocytes
   D. all of the above

3. An antigen is:
 • A. any substance capable of eliciting an immune response
   B. the substrate in the body that reacts to a foreign substance
   C. always a protein
   D. the "second wave" of host defense

4. T-cells are:
   A. the primary cells of cell-mediated immunity
   B. involved in almost all types of adaptive immune reactions
 • C. both A & B
   D. none of the above

5. A patient with a history of repeated bacterial infections is most likely to have a defect in their:
   A. cell-mediated immunity
 • B. humoral mediated immune response

   C. innate immunity
   D. all of the above

6. Immune deficiencies are commonly associated with:
   A. diabetes
   B. alcoholism
   C. burns
 • D. all of the above

7. HIV disease primarily affects:
   A. T8 killer cells
   B. memory lymphocytes
 • C. T4 helper cells
   D. B lymphocytes

8. Following an exposure to HIV infected body fluid, AZT is most effective if given:
   A. within 48-72 hours of exposure
 • B. within 4 hours of exposure
   C. within 1 hour of exposure
   D. none of the above

9. The most effective nursing measure in the prevention of nosocomial infections is:
   A. appropriate patient isolation
   B. strict adherence to sterile technique
   C. use of universal precautions
 • D. frequent handwashing

10. During an arterial line insertion, health care workers should take the following precautions:
 • A. gown, gloves, mask, protective eye wear
   B. gown, gloves, mask
   C. gloves, mask
   D. gloves, mask, protective eyewear